GETTING PAST THE PAIN

THE PAIN Making Sense of Life's Darkness

To my parents,
Elsie Mae and Hillard Witt,
who shared sixty-four years of marriage,
and who taught me not to fear the dark

Getting Past the Pain

Making Sense of Life's Darkness

William Powell Tuck

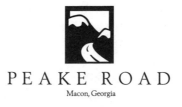

PEAKE ROAD
Macon, Georgia

ISBN 1-57312-158-4

Getting Past the Pain
Making Sense of Life's Darkness

William Powell Tuck
Copyright © 1997
Peake Road

6316 Peake Road
Macon, Georgia 31210-3960
1-800-747-3016
Peake Road is an imprint of
Smyth & Helwys Publishing, Inc.

From "Questions about Darkness," *Proclaim,* January-March 1988.
© Copyright 1987. The Sunday School Board of the Southern
Baptist Convention. All rights reserved. Used by permission.

Library of Congress Cataloging–in–Publication Data
Tuck, William Powell, 1934-
    Getting past the pain: making sense of life's darkness/
William Powell Tuck.
    Includes bibliographical references.
    x + 134 pp.   6" x 9" (15 x 23 cm.)
    ISBN 1-57312-158-4   (alk. paper)
    1. Pain—Religious aspects—Christianity.
    2. Suffering—Religious aspects—Christianity.
    3. Sin. 4. Good and evil.
    5. Encouragement—Religious aspects—Christianity.
    6. Hope—Religious aspects—Christianity.
    I. Title.
    BV4909.T83   1997
    248.8'6—dc21   97-6080
                                          CIP

Contents

Foreword

Spiritual edification awaits you as you read this book of essays on human suffering in the dark experiences that either you face now or sooner or later will face. The word "edification" has fallen into disuse in daily conversation, even in the fellowship of our churches. It has become overgrown with weeds of neglect. Yet its faraway, quaint sound faintly alerts our sleeping spirits to arise and watch and pray lest we enter into temptation. Our neglect of edification of our own lives in the disciplines of the Christian faith may well explain much of the conflict that besets many churches and denominations.

Edification simply means to build up the quality of the fellowship of Christians. It is the opposite of "tearing one another down," "putting one another down," "shattering each other apart." Edification of people in times of despair, the burden of sin, the multiplicity of suffering, the threat and/or crisis of suicide, the burdens of responsibility, the realities of facing and accepting death—this is the stuff of which William Tuck's book is made.

Tuck is committed to a ministry of encouragement to his readers. He is concerned that you and I have a profound sense of the presence of God as the source of serenity and hope in our times of darkness. He quietly reasons with us in our proneness to want easy answers to the dark mysteries that beset us. He, as the good shepherd he is, nudges, prods, and commands us to cease and desist when we move toward shallow optimism, cynicism, and the projection of blame for our plight upon God. He enables us to face squarely who God is in Jesus Christ when we ascribe to God actions for which we would imprison a person as a brutal criminal were he or she to do such things. To the contrary, Tuck portrays God in Christ as sharing with us the dark times of our lives as we live them out within the limits of humanity. He inspires us to put our suffering to use, to exercise the ingenuity inspired by God's challenging presence to devise moral and spiritual uses of dark things.

William Tuck presents "eyewitness accounts" of people who have struggled in unimaginably dark situations of life. He presents "living

human documents" from the autobiographies and biographies of wit-
nesses—even martyrs—both to formulate and to demonstrate his
convictions. From the student's or pastor's point of view, this book is a
storehouse of well-documented testimonies of people under the stress
of dark times in their lives.

I had the privilege of having William Tuck as my pastor when my
family and I went through some very dark and troubling times of illness and perplexity. His steadfast ministry to us caused me to know
with what integrity he speaks in these pages. Furthermore, I served as
a staff member of our church during some dark days of the life of our
church. He came to us after our building had burned down, after we
had lost our pastor, and while we were meeting in borrowed buildings.
He saw us through dark times both for us and for himself. Consequently, the first-handedness of these documents gives them the
authenticity of a writer who knows from experience whereof he speaks.
I commend his book to you wholeheartedly and with great gratitude
to William Tuck.

Wayne E. Oates

Preface

In an article long lost to me, I copied a line from W. B. J. Martin about the demise of liberal theology.

> As far as I can see, it languished because it paid more attention to method than to content. . . . It paid insufficient attention to the dark side of life, those underground factors which, although not easily accessible to reason, are nevertheless the nourishment of life.

The words, "it paid insufficient attention to the dark side of life," leaped out at me. No theology can survive that ignores the dark side of life. I had rather think, speak, or write about the joys and happiness, fun and humor of life, because everyone's life would be empty without them. But life is not filled only with sunshine. Dark, difficult days are also a part of the fabric of life's tapestry. We all wish it were not so, but the dark is as real as the light.

Questions about the darkness—sin, burdens, suffering, AIDS, suicide, aging, and death—raise huge question marks about life's purpose, God's love and care, our responsibility for our actions and what others do, and the plain fairness or unfairness of life.

- What causes a person to sin?
- Can I simply do anything I want without concern for others?
- Why is there so much pain and suffering in life?
- Should Christians be spared pain and agony?
- Why do good, kind people have to bear unspeakable burdens?
- Why does God not prevent suicide, war, and disease?
- Why does a good God permit suffering and allow death?
- Why do we have to die?
- Do we live after death, or is the grave the end?
- Is there a God and, if so, where?
- Why does God hide God's face and not answer our questions?

Questions, often unanswerable questions, leap to our mind and lips. These questions arise out of the dark places of life. They are your questions and mine. We long—even cry—for an answer. "Oh God, are you there?" In these pages I have not denied the questions about the dark, but I have attempted to listen to these haunting questions and respond as honestly as I can. My struggle has helped me. I hope you will find some source of encouragement in these pages as well. I have not attempted to give the answer because I cannot, and frankly, I don't think anyone can. But in struggling in the dark, we can sense the pulsebeat of the God who is there with us in the darkness.

I want to thank Wayne Oates for reading my manuscript and giving me his encouragement, support, and critical counsel. He has been a pastor friend to me on many a dark day. I owe a real debt to Carolyn Stice, my former secretary, who typed these pages through numerous drafts, always doing so with graciousness and a supportive spirit. I also want to thank Marie Barkley, my secretary, for her faithful assistance in seeing this work brought to its finished state. Ida Helm willingly read the entire manuscript and offered her critical counsel. Special thanks also to Helen Crenshaw and Bill Tubbs who provided invaluable technical assistance in the final stages. I am appreciative of all that these persons have contributed.

Acknowledging the Darkness

The Old Testament begins with darkness, and the last of the Gospels ends with it. "Darkness was upon the face of the deep," Genesis says. Darkness was where it all started. Before darkness, there had never been anything other than darkness, void and without form.

At the end of John, the disciples go out fishing on the Sea of Tiberias. It is night. They have no luck. Their nets are empty. Then they spot somebody standing on the beach. At first they don't see who it is in the darkness. It is Jesus.

The darkness of Genesis is broken by God in great majesty speaking the word of creation. "Let there be light!" That's all it took.

The darkness of John is broken by the flicker of a charcoal fire on the sand. Jesus has made it. He cooks some fish on it for his old friends' breakfast. On the horizon there are the first pale traces of the sun getting ready to rise.

All the genius and glory of God are somehow represented by these two scenes, not to mention what Saint Paul calls God's foolishness.

Frederick Buechner
Listening to Your Life[1]

The night has many faces. Some of the faces are hostile, but sometimes the night may even take on a friendly pose. James Agee, in his book entitled *A Death in the Family*, pictures a young boy as he is reflecting on the approaching darkness of the night. As he sees the night coming, he remarks:

Gentle, gentle dark. My darkness. Do you listen? Oh, are you hallowed, all one taking ear? My darkness. Do you watch me? Oh, are you rounded, all one guardian eye? O gentlest dark. Gentlest, gentlest night. My darkness. My dear darkness. Under your shelter all things come and go. . . . You come to us once each day and never a day rises into brightness but you stand behind it; you are upon us, you overwhelm us all each night. It is you who releases from work, who brings parted families and friends together, and people for a little while are calm and free, and all at ease together; but before long, before long, all are brought down silent and motionless. Under your sheltering, your great sheltering darkness. And all through that silence you walked as if none but you had ever breathed or ever dreamed, had ever been. . . . Tell me your secrets; you can trust me. Come near. Come very near.[2]

But when the darkness does come near the young boy, it ceases to be friendly to him, and he begins to cry for his father to come and assist him in the night. He, too, found that the night was not always gentle and the darkness was not always friendly.

The Threatening Darkness

Sometimes the darkness of the night seems to overwhelm and threaten us. The book of Job pictures its hero as living in a kind of Shangri-la where everything in his life seemed to be comfortable and secure. But, then, illness fell upon his family, and death struck them. His crops began to fail. Enemies plundered his home and property, and he came down with a dread disease. Job, who represents every man and woman, cried out, "I waited for the light, but darkness came. I cried out to you, but you did not answer me. Why do you hide your face from me?"

Eugene O'Neill expressed in a powerful drama the feeling of many. people who are caught within the darkness of life today. The title itself, *A Long Day's Journey into Night,* expresses the frustration of many. The Tyrone family, around whom the play centers, lives in a personal world filled with darkness. The play focuses on personal tragedy in its beginning and ends in tragedy as none of the family members find an answer in their darkness. They move further into the darkness of their own night.

Many people have struggled in their own darkness and have wondered where God was. Where was light out of the dark? Where was the answer? A man said to me one time: "Pastor, it would be very easy for me to be an atheist in this kind of world, because, frankly, I don't know where God is a lot of the time." His problems seemed so immense, and God did not seem to be there. A soldier looked up at his chaplain during a fierce battle and exclaimed, "You know what's wrong, chaplain? You know why we are fighting and dying all over the world all of the time? Your God has let us down. He simply has let us down." He, too, walked in darkness.

As a young pastor, I walked into the home of a church family and tried to help the members as they struggled with the sad news that the baby who had just been born into their family had Down's Syndrome. How could they face the darkness of uncertainty that had enveloped them? What do you say to the parents of a young teenage boy who was a star basketball player in high school and had received a full scholarship to attend his state university but was gunned down by some unknown assailants one night as he was walking home? Darkness enveloped that family. I have walked with people through dark valleys when they were overtaken by an illness that lingered on and on. Illness may have struck either a parent or a child who could not live and could not die, but simply vegetated. They cried out from their darkness, "Where is God?" I remember walking the path toward a cemetery with the parents of a sixteen-year-old girl who had a cerebral hemorrhage and lingered for a week, and then, died. They cried out from the darkness of their grief and asked, "God, where are you?"

Four centuries ago Sir John Hawkins christened his ship and set sail for Africa. He sailed along the coast of Africa and captured black natives. He put them in chains, took them aboard his ship, and brought them to his homeland to be sold into slavery. This "noble man" christened his slave ship, *Jesus*. Where was God in that kind of darkness?

There is darkness within our world, and we need to be honest enough to admit it. If we see no darkness, we have not lived very long, or our eyes are closed to the world around us. I want us to look at some of the dark places of life and examine the issues of sin, burdens, suffering, AIDS, suicide, pain, and death. Darkness raises questions that sometimes we want to avoid. We pretend they do not exist, or we ignore them. I want us to see if there is some light from God that can shine within the darkness to give us direction and hope when these struggles come upon us.

When God Seems Hidden

First, let's be open and honest and admit that sometimes God does seem to be hidden. If you have never experienced in some way or another the hiddenness of God in your life, then you are very unusual. The Scriptures declare that God both conceals God's self as well as reveals God's self. Some people attempt to face the difficulties of life by asserting that they are an illusion. "Sin, pain, suffering, and death do not exist," they state. But I have great difficulty with that view. Walk with me into any cancer ward and then tell me that pain and death are illusions, especially when the one suffering is your child, husband, wife, or parent. No, suffering, pain, grief, and death are not illusions; they are real. They are a part of our world.

Others answer the dilemma by saying that we are thrown back upon our own individual resources to face whatever comes. We can expect no help from anyone else, especially not from some divine being. We believe that only our own resources can sustain us. These voices cry out and ask, "Where was your God when the President was assassinated?" "Where was God when a senator was assassinated?" "Where was God when a governor was gunned down?" "Where was God when babies or old women were raped?" "Where was God in the midst of all of this pain?" When we see all that has happened in our world, these exponents assert that only our own resources will enable us to survive.

A book entitled *Night*, written by a German author named Elie Wiesel, relates the author's experience in one of the worst German concentration camps of World War II. He saw his own sister led off to a gas chamber and put to death. Here are his words as he reflected on that experience:

> Never shall I forget that night, the first night in camp, which has turned my life into one long night, seven times cursed and seven times sealed. Never shall I forget that smoke. Never shall I forget the little faces of the children, whose bodies I saw turned into wreaths of smoke beneath a silent blue sky. Never shall I forget those flames which consumed my faith forever. Never shall I forget that nocturnal silence which deprived me for all eternity of the desire to live. Never shall I forget those moments which murdered my God and my soul and turned my dreams to dust. Never shall I forget those things even if I am condemned to live as God Himself. Never.[3]

Here was a man whose experiences in the German concentration camps caused him to lose his faith in God. He lost his family, his faith, and everything worthwhile to him. For him, God was hidden and has continued to remain hidden. To him, God lingered in the darkness, and the darkness of night promised no dawn for him.

There have been dark moments in your life as well. They may not have been as dark as Wiesel's, but dark, nevertheless. For you, darkness might take the form of failure or disappointment. Some persons have known the darkness of the loss of a job, a broken romance, pain, suffering, grief, or death. Who among us has not known some kind of dark moment in which God's spirit seemed hidden from us, and we cried, "God show me your face in the midst of all this darkness." God seems far from us.

Winter in the Heart

In his book, *A Cry of Absence,* Martin Marty wrote about the elusive presence of God in his own experience of grief at the death of his wife. "Not every believer can move easily into the rhythms of country-and-western Christianity with its foot-stomping, exuberant styles."[4] His experience had been a "winter in the heart" as he grappled with pain, loss, and death.

The writer of Psalm 88 raised this kind of question out of his own struggles. Some of the Israelites had been taken captive to Babylonia. They were away from their homeland, away from their home, their place of worship, the Temple, and everything that was dear to them. They were cast into their enemies' land and made slaves. Out of their despair, they cried out to God and asked, "God, where are you? Do you not care?" Some of them had been to the abyss of life and believed that life was without meaning, without hope, and without direction. They reached out to see if God were present in this strange land and if God really cared for them at all.

Some of those who were in the darkest of nights saw a star, some glimmer of hope. Some slowly began to realize that through their suffering, they had developed sympathy for others. Out of their tragedy, they developed a new vision of hope. Some of them, out of the worst kinds of circumstances of life, began to build a deep and lasting faith. Some discovered a new awareness that God could be worshiped anywhere. Others found new direction for their life and found hope for the future in the midst of all their suffering.

In a modern-day setting, the cartoon character Snoopy is lying on top of his doghouse. Charlie Brown comes by and exclaims, "Huh, some beagle scout you are. You got lost in the woods. Don't you know that 'N' on the compass stands for north?" Snoopy muses to himself. "Oh, I thought that meant nowhere." A lot of folks who have experienced the dark have felt that God was nowhere to be found. God seemed nowhere near. Their experience was of a God that remained hidden to them.

God's Presence

Note that the Scriptures reveal that God is in the darkness as well as in the light. God is not with us just when it is light, but God is also with us in the darkness. Sometimes darkness may be friendly; it is not always hostile. In fact, you and I could not exist very well without darkness. The dark gives us opportunity to rest and let our bodies be restored. During darkness God gives us the gift of sleep so we can have opportunity for rest and restoration. Some animals, such as mice, are active mostly at night. Certain birds migrate at night. Some birds sing at night. Some insects are busy only at night.

Several years ago I saw a television special that depicted a new form of life that exists at the lowest depths of the oceans, where no human eye has ever seen, and where light never reaches. Life exists there even in complete darkness. Darkness is a part of life. Living goes on in the darkness.

James G. Emerson, in his book, *Suffering: Its Meaning and Ministry*, states that the real question is not "Why does God permit suffering?" "The real issue is that God wishes for us the ultimate experience of being truly creative. That experience must include the darkness—the shadow." He continues his thought with this insight:

> The reality of pain and the presence of evil are not evidence against God, but evidence for the ground of all our living. Once again, we find that the reality of the cross is the evidence that when we suffer, God suffers with us. God is in the shadow. If God is in the suffering, too, how can we blame God? We must live with the shadow.[5]

In the year 1910, a ship named *Republic* was sinking and radioed for help. Another ship, the *Baltic*, had gone to see if it could rescue the passengers from the sinking vessel, but the fog was so heavy the crew members were not able to locate the ship. They searched for the ship in the fog and sounded their mournful whistle, but there was no response. Then, as darkness of the night settled on the ocean, the light of the ship *Republic* could be seen. Then, the *Baltic* moved closer for the rescue. In this instance, the darkness helped the search. There are times when darkness may be our friend.

The Scriptures affirm that even in the darkest of moments or the dreariest of days, God is present with us in the darkness. The psalmist reminds us that to God the darkness and the light are the same (Ps 139:12). God is present in both. Darkness does not separate us from God's presence. Some of us look for God only in the lovely, beautiful places of life. But God is present in all of life. We cannot flee or hide from God's presence. God is present not only in the sunshine but in the darkness, in the thorn as well as in the rose, in the earthquake as well as in the lilies of the field, in the snowstorm as well as in the spring crops, in famine as well as in plenty, in defeat as well as in victory.

As the psalmist declared,

> Where can I go from your spirit? Or where can I flee from your presence? If I ascend to heaven, you are there; if I make my bed in Sheol, you are there; . . . Even the darkness is not dark to you; the night is as bright as the day, for darkness is as light to you. (Ps 139:7-8, 12)

There is a powerful passage in Exodus 20:21 that describes Moses' encounter with God in the darkness on top of Mount Sinai. "The people stood at a distance, while Moses drew near to the thick darkness where God was." All the rest of the people waited while Moses met God in the darkness. But the Scriptures are clear—God was in the darkness.

Blaise Pascal once observed that "a religion which does not affirm that God is hidden is not true. *Vere tu es Deus absconditas!*" The Hebrew-Christian faith attests that God reveals God's self. But in the same breath the Scriptures declare, "Truly you are a God who hides himself!" (Isa 45:15). God is always beyond our grasp even when God has disclosed God's self. Even in divine revelation, God remains hidden. Samuel Terrien noted,

> In biblical faith, human beings discern that presence is a surging which soon vanishes and leaves in its disappearance an absence that has been overcome. It is neither absolute nor eternal but elusive and fragile, even and especially when human beings seek to prolong it in the form of cults. The collective act of worship seems to be both the

indispensable vehicle of presence and its destroyer. It is when presence escapes man's grasp that it surges, survives, or returns. It is also
when human beings meet in social responsibility that presence,
once vanished, is heard.[6]

Learning from Experiences

Sometimes you and I may learn more about God in the darkness than
we do in the light. Many of us who have lived in the light of comfort
and joy sometimes have difficulty experiencing God when we enter
the dark moments of our lives. But there are some people who have
experienced the reality of God's presence in the dark places of life in
ways that they never would have known otherwise.

A woman possessed a beautiful voice, but, as her professor of
music listened to her sing one day, he said to a colleague, "She is a
magnificent singer. And yet there is something lacking in her singing.
Life has been too kind to her. But if one day it happened that someone broke her heart, she would be the finest singer in Europe!" That is
a rather harsh thing to say, but there is a ring of reality in that
statement.

Sometimes we are not truly sympathetic until we ourselves have
suffered. Sometimes we are not able to comfort another until we have
known discomfort and grief. We can never be courageous until we
ourselves have known cowardliness. We may not understand true faith
until we have struggled with our own disbelief. Sometimes out of our
own pain comes concern, grace, and caring for other people. When
we walk into the darkness of the holy of holies of our own "dark night
of the soul," we are ultimately drawn closer to God.

I remember the first time I read a powerful statement in one of
James Stewart's books. He noted that usually the great sufferers in life
have not been the skeptics. Instead, the great sufferers in life have been
the great saints. The spectators who observe the great sufferers have
been the skeptics. Many who have gone through periods of agony and
difficulty have become the most saintly of people. "Indeed, the fact is
that it is the world's greatest sufferers who have produced the most
shining examples of unconquerable faith."[7]

Jacob wrestled in a creekbed gorge at Kedron in the darkness of
the night trying to find God. In his encounter with God that night,
his name was changed from Jacob to Israel. He became the founder of

a great nation. In that dark night he was remade and renamed. Moses wrestled with God in a wilderness place, and then moved into the thick darkness to meet God. When he came down from Mount Sinai, out of that darkness, he did not know that his countenance was shining. Jeremiah wrestled with God in his own agony, suffering, pain, rejection, failure, and ridicule. Out of all his agony, he was drawn closer to the power and presence of God, and he had an effect upon a whole nation. Elijah crawled into a cave mourning, groaning, weeping, and bemoaning his state. Out of his own chastisement, God spoke softly to him. God raised Elijah out of suffering to serve more effectively. Even Jesus wrestled with himself in the Garden of Gethsemane and cried that his cup of suffering might pass from him.

Finding God

Many great souls have wrestled in the darkness of their experiences to find God, and out of that darkness, they have found the reality of God's presence that has sustained them. They have become stronger men and women, not weaker persons, because of the struggle. Oh, there are some who turn away from God in the darkness, but more have turned toward God than away, and their lives have been transformed.

In Pilqrim's Progress, Christian needs help and he turns to Evangelist and asks for guidance on his journey toward the Celestial City. Evangelist points him toward the way and asks, "Do you see yonder wicket-gate?" Christian looks off in the distance and replies, "No." Evangelist points again and asks, "Do you see yonder shining light?" Christian peers off into the darkness and finally sees a spot that does not seem to be as dark as the rest of the darkness, and he says, "I think I do." "Keep that light in your eye," Evangelist states. "And go up directly thereto, so shall thou see the gate."

In the midst of the darkness we are able to move toward that light, whether that light comes from the support of a friend or the encouragement of a neighbor or the prayers of the church. As we move toward that light, the gate becomes more visible, the path more apparent, and the way more sure. But we must move toward the light we have. And we have to walk with the assurance that God is there with us in the darkness, as well as in the light that lies before us.

When I was a seminary student, one of my professors auto-graphed for me a book he had published. He wrote this inscription in it: *Sursum Corda*. It had been quite a while since I had studied Latin, so it was hard to figure out. But I discovered it means, "Lift up your heads." It was drawn from the passage that reads: "Lift up your heads; for your redemption draweth nigh" (Luke 21:28 KJV). As Christians, we have the promise that in the darkest moment of life, we can lift up our heads. Remember, God is there with us in the darkness, and God is pointing us toward the light that sustains us. I like the understanding we can draw from the Greek word, *anthropos*, which means "man." *Anthropos*, in its root form, means "the creature that looks up." Do not look down into the darkness that surrounds you. Don't just look around in the gloom. Look up. Lift up your heart with the assurance that God is there to sustain you and take you safely through the darkness to the light beyond.

Helping Others

When you come to those dark moments in life, remember to give whatever assistance you can to others you meet in the darkness. The light you offer to others in the darkness can make a difference in their lives as they try to walk through that darkness.

It is easy to curse the darkness. It is easy to gripe about the darkness, talk about it, and complain about it. There are dark nights of all kinds. We experience dark nights of disappointment and sorrow, dark nights of indifference and pain, dark nights of discouragement and opposition. We may have known dark nights of doubt and anxiety, persecution and bewilderment, rejection and loneliness, depression and isolation. If we sense the light of only one star in the darkest of nights, that one pale light can provide illumination to our path and direction for our journey. That faint light encourages us, and we travel on toward more light. And, as we journey, we seek to offer light to others from our light, even if it is faint, that this light might offer some illumination to others for whom the night is darker. You and I may not be able to eliminate all the darkness with our light. We may not be able to remove all the pain, problems, or difficulties, but we can lift up our light wherever we are to help others as they struggle along the way with us.

As director of the United Farm Workers, Cesar Chavez labored hard to improve conditions for the migrant workers over the years. He tells about an experience he had when he was about fourteen years old. He and his family were migrating as they usually did, trying to find enough farm work to give themselves a livable income. One day, he said, they went into a restaurant to eat. A sign was posted that read, "Whites Only." Being Mexicans, they were hoping they could be served. They sat down at a table. A waitress gave them a menu and went back to get the water for their table. The owner of the restaurant chastised her for having seated them. He told her to throw them out or he would fire her. She had to come back to the table and tell them, "I'm sorry, I can't serve you. You have to leave." As the family got up and walked away, Cesar walked over to the owner of the restaurant. He said he could stand it no longer, and although he was only a fourteen-year-old boy, he felt he had to speak. His family called to him to come, but he said, "I have to speak up someday and it's going to be today." He went over to the boss and asked, "Why do you have to treat people like that? Any man who behaves like you do is not even a human being." The man cursed him and said, "G'wan, get out of here." But he said from that moment on, he was determined to lift his voice against the darkness of prejudice.

We may be only one small voice whispering in the dark, but that can be a beginning. Soon that voice may be joined with another and another and another. Your voice and mine can be voices that are raised against the injustice, ignorance, suffering, and pain in the world to guide people out of the darkness into the light of the way of Christ.

The Light Shines

The Scriptures tell us that the darkness has not mastered the light. The darkness has not overcome the light. The darkness has not overtaken it. It has not extinguished the light. The light that Christ brought into the world is a light that emanates from the very presence of God. This light has not been mastered and has not been overcome. It continues to illuminate the world and guide people in the way of goodness and righteousness. As long as that light is shinning, justice, righteousness, and goodness shall continue to be accomplished in the world. As long as that light sends its beam shining into the world, it offers guidance along the pathway of life.

Viktor Frankl's book, *Man's Search for Meaning*, describes the experience he had in one of the German concentration camps in

World War II. One day while he was digging in a trench, he was thinking about his wife and all the misery he was enduring. Here are his own words:

> The dawn was gray around us, gray was the sky above; gray was the snow in the pale light of dawn, gray the rags in which my fellow prisoners were clad, and gray their faces. I was again conversing silently with my wife, or perhaps I was struggling to find the reason for my suffering, my slow dying. In a last violent protest against the hopelessness of an imminent death, I sensed my spirit piercing through the enveloping gloom. I felt it transcend that hopeless, meaningless world, and from somewhere I heard a victorious "Yes" in answer to my question of the existence of an ultimate purpose. At that moment a light was lit in a distant farmhouse, which stood on the horizon as if painted there, in the midst of the miserable gray of the dawning of morning in Bavaria. "*Et lux in tenebris lucet*—and the light shineth in the darkness."[8]

In the darkness of his prison camp, and in the worst circumstances of his life, Frankl saw in the distance a morning light in a farmhouse. For him, that light offered hope and encouragement. It reminded him of an even greater light—the presence of God. In the darkest moment in your life and in my life, we have the assurance that God is there with the light of the divine presence to guide us. The powers of evil, the powers of pain, the powers of death cannot conquer it. The light of God's presence has not been mastered. It will continue to burn. Darkness cannot put out the glow of its flame.

Several years ago in our country, a young boy and his sister had gone on a tour down into the depths of a cavern. After they had descended a great distance, they reached a point in the tour, as they do in most cavern tours, where the lights were turned off to emphasize the absolute blackness there. The young girl had not expected the light to go out and cried out. Her brother reached over and took her hand and reassured her as he said, "Don't cry, little sister. There is somebody here who knows how to turn on the lights." We don't have to be afraid. There is one who is the Light. It is Jesus Christ, our Lord. In the darkest moment of any night or day, be assured that he is there, and he knows how to turn on the lights.

Notes

[1]Frederick Buechner, *Listening to Your Life*, comp. George Connor (San Francisco: Harper-Collins, 1992) 153-54.

[2]James Agee, *A Death in the Family* (New York: Grossett & Dunlap, 1957) 65-67.

[3]Elie Wiesel, *Night* (New York: Avon Books, 1960) 9.

[4]Martin Marty, *A Cry of Absence* (San Francisco: Harper & Row, 1983) 5.

[5]James G. Emerson, *Suffering: Its Meaning and Ministry* (Nashville: Abingdon Press, 1986) 131.

[6]Samuel Terrien, *The Elusive Presence* (San Francisco: Harper & Row, 1983) 476.

[7]James S. Stewart, *The Strong Name* (New York: Charles Scribner's Sons, 1941) 153.

[8]Viktor Frank, *Man's Search for Meaning* (New York: Washington Square Press, 1963) 63-64.

Struggling in the Darkness

Sin

"Sin" is a word that is vanishing from our culture's vocabulary now. The editors of dictionaries have not yet ruled it archaic and restricted it to the limbo of unabridged editions. Yet the word "sin" is a step into an older language that Americans passively retain but do not actively use outside church. To those who do not go to church, "sin" is a code word for the whole mess of superstition that the modern world has thrown off.

William S. Stafford
Disordered Loves
Healing the Seven Deadly Sins[1]

Sin is not a private transaction between the sinner and God. Humanity always crowds the audience-room when God holds court. We must democratize the conception of God; then the definition of sin will become more realistic.

We love and serve God when we love and serve our fellows, whom he loves and in whom he lives. We rebel against God and repudiate his will when we set our profit and ambition above the welfare of our fellows and above the Kingdom of God which binds them together.

Walter Rauschenbusch
A Theology for the Social Gospel[2]

I believe the postmodern world will require a different theology, and I have tried to suggest where that theology must come from and what it will be. But I believe that such a theology cannot be successfully formulated unless the modern liberal legacy is appropriated and incorporated. Only a theology that has taken the modern age seriously will be able to take seriously what is coming next. No one can move beyond the secular city who has not first passed through it.

Harvey Cox
Religion in the Secular City[3]

A young boy brought his report card home. He had received rather low marks in conduct. When his father asked him about his low marks, he replied, "But Dad, conduct is my hardest subject." And so it is for all of us. Conduct is really our hardest subject in life. There are many who want to say that our conduct—how we live and how we act—is simply left up to us. Morality is fluid, they say. It is in motion. There is no such thing as right and wrong. Each decides for himself or herself what is right or wrong.

Assuming a Special Knowledge of God

John was no stranger to this kind of attitude regarding right and wrong. He penned his small epistle to confront those who wanted to live by the same approach in his day (see 1 John 1:5-10). John was dealing with a group of people called the Gnostics. The Gnostics believed that they had a "special knowledge" about God and life, and, therefore, they lived on a level superior to others. They claimed that either they had not sinned at all or they had no responsibility for their sins, because they lived above them. John was writing to them about the reality of sin and the darkness that sin brings within one's life.

Jesus was confronted by some religious leaders in his day who attempted to make rules and regulations about life exact and formalized. All one had to do was to abide by the rule book. If they did, their relationship with God would be alright. But that approach got difficult very early, because those who drew up the rule book began to add footnotes to their regulations and then footnotes to the footnotes.

Some of the rabbinical schools in the day of Jesus began to split hairs over whether or not a woman was bearing a burden if she stuck a needle in her dress when she was sewing. If a person traveled more than a prescribed distance from his home on the Sabbath, he was committing a sin. They even debated whether or not one could eat an egg that was laid on the Sabbath. We still have those today who want to legitimize morality for us. They want to prescribe morality and tell us what to do. We have to follow their morality code. The legalists are still with us today.

Allowing Conscience to Be Our Guide

But, then, there are those who want to be on the other end of the moral scale and say, "Well, just let me make my own decisions. I will decide. My conscience will determine what is right and wrong for me. I do not need any church, any God, anybody telling me how I should live or how I should act." I guess my problem with that approach is that I am troubled with some people's untroubled consciences. Some people's consciences will let them do anything in any place or at any time.

There was a time when some consciences said, "It's ok to make human sacrifices," and they did. Neither Hitler nor the German soldiers involved in Nazism let their conscience stop them from annihilating six million Jews. Today in China, parents are permitted to have only one child. If a couple has more than one child, they lose their tax exemptions and may be penalized in other ways. Since a male child is preferred, often the female child is killed, and the parents wait until a male child is born to keep the baby. I am very troubled by those who want to say, "I will let my conscience be my guide," because the history of the world is filled with pages stained by blood based on individual decisions about right and wrong.

Not Accepting Responsibility

There is no question in my mind that some guidelines are essential for meaningful living. Yet, like the early Gnostics, we want to cry out and say, "I am not responsible for the sins of society. I am not responsible for my own sin. I am really free from blame."

You may occasionally read the cartoon in the daily newspaper called the "Family Circus." That cartoon often depicts an "invisible" figure. This figure usually appears in the background. The mother or father will ask the children if they have done something. They might be asked, for example, if they have left their father's paintbrush on top of the open can to dry, or if they have left his tools in the woods, or if they have put their fingerprints on the wall. Each time, when they are reprimanded for various things, they reply, "Not me." This "invisible" figure is seen in each of these pieces as symbolizing another person called "Not me."

In our society today some of us almost always want to say "not me." We point to someone else for the blame. We blame heredity. We blame the environment. We blame illness. We blame circumstances or emotions. It is always someone else's fault. We do this individually, and we do this as a nation. You see it all the time in politics. "It was the previous administration that caused this problem." We continuously pass on our faults to another. Some parents even place the blame for their actions on their children. The attempt at disassociation is a favorite idea of Harry Stack Sullivan. The "not-me" mode is, according to Sullivan, "part of the very 'private mode' of living, but . . . it manifests itself at various times in the life of everyone after childhood—or of nearly everyone."[4]

In a "Peanuts" cartoon, Lucy walks up to Charlie Brown and says to him, "I want to talk to you, Charlie Brown. As your sister's consulting psychiatrist, I must put the blame for her fears on you." "On me?" Charlie Brown responds. "Each generation," Lucy continues, "must be able to blame the previous generation for its problems. It doesn't solve anything. But it makes us all feel better!" Each wants to blame another for what he or she is. This does not mean that heredity, the environment, or circumstances have nothing to do with who and what we are. They are a significant part. But these factors do not remove our own responsibility for whom we have become.

Who's Responsible for My Sins?

Karl Menninger, who is not a practicing theologian, but a psychiatrist, wrote a book entitled, *Whatever Became of Sin?* In that book, he focuses on the reality of sin in the behavior of people. Although he is well aware of the factors that constitute and influence a person's background, he calls for an awareness of personal responsibility in moral values. We can't always blame circumstances and others for our present state. Our sense of guilt, anxious mind, loss of direction, and confusion of thought are rooted in our need for the recognition of sin. He reminds us that sometimes the fault with our present state is a result of the sin within us.

In his book *On Not Leaving It to the Snake*, Harvey Cox, a theologian at Harvard University, begins discussion with Adam and Eve who would not take responsibility for their own sins. They blamed the snake. Down through the centuries, individuals have constantly blamed other "snakes" for their problems by refusing to take responsibility for their own sense of sinfulness. We always believe that someone or something else has caused our problems. The fault always lies elsewhere.

A noted theologian, Paul Tillich, penned these words:

> Have the men of our time still a feeling of the meaning of sin? Do
> they, and do we, still realize that sin does not mean an immoral act,
> that "sin," should never be used in the plural, and that not our sins,
> but rather our sin is the great, all-pervading problem of our life? . . .
> To be in the state of sin is to be in the state of separation.

Separation, he states, may be from one's fellowman, from one's own
true self, or from our God. Tillich continues,

> But there is a mysterious fact about the great words of our religious
> tradition: they cannot be replaced. All attempts to make substitu-
> tions, including those I have tried myself, have failed to convey the
> reality that was to be expressed; they have led to shallow and impo-
> tent talk. There are no substitutes for words like "sin," and "grace."[5]

Sin is that which separates us, Tillich says, from ourselves, from
God, and from others. Sin is the fragmentation that destroys relationship. Sin, in its widest sense, is not just our individual sins. It is our
sense of sinfulness—our "godalmightiness." Sin is an attempt to assert
our "myness." This is our way of saying, "I want to take control of my
life, without any sense of needing God. I am totally in control. I am
the master of my fate, the captain of my soul. I do not need others nor
God."

A contemporary German theologian, Wolfhart Pannenberg, said
that one of the mistakes of the church is separating the forgiveness of
sins from baptism. He declares that the Scriptures are clear in showing
that sin and the forgiveness of sins are a matter of death and life. In
the early church, the connection between baptism and the death and
resurrection of Christ was clear to candidates.[6] Pannenberg is a member of the Reformed Church tradition where baptism by immersion is
not practiced. Protestants who practice believer's baptism have not lost
the original symbolism. When a person is led into the baptistery, and
he or she is lowered under the water, death to the old way of sin is
symbolized. The person is raised, as Christ was from the grave, to walk
in newness of life with him.

Sin is the reality that leads, the Scriptures declare, to death. Sin, in
all of its seriousness, creates death within our authentic self, death in
our relationship with other people, and most profoundly, it has separated us from God. The Scriptures are very clear about the darkness of

sin. "For the wages of sin is death" (Rom 6:23). Sin threatens our sense of life's meaning, and our self-centeredness results in death. Death is the consequence of a meaningless life that has lost its sense of direction and purpose.

The Loss of Innocence

I am too old to talk about being innocent, and, if you can read this, so are you. I can remember, and you can too, when we had some sense of innocence. I can remember when I didn't know what divorce was. I can recall a time before I knew what war, or murder, or death was. I can remember when I didn't know what adultery was. All of these were totally unknown to me. I was a child, and I was completely innocent of such knowledge. But I am too old, and I have committed too many sins not to believe in the reality of sin.

I recall one of the first times in my conscious life when I knew I had done something that I really should not have done. I knew what I was doing. I knew I was doing it against my parents' desires. Most of all, I had an aching feeling that I didn't think even God wanted me to do it, but I did it anyway. I do not deny the reality of sin because I know that I am a sinner. I have worked, counseled, and talked with too many other people not to know that we are all sinners. "If we claim to be sinless, we are self-deceived and strangers to the truth" (1 John 1:8 NEB). John tells us that if we pretend we have no sin or if we attempt to deny our sin, then we make God a liar. God has spoken about the reality of sin within our world. It is here. We cannot pretend to be innocent. When we sin, we hurt ourselves, others, and ultimately, God.

The Freedom to Choose

God has created the kind of universe in which sin is possible. When we sin, God doesn't reach over and say, "Ah, I saw you do that, and I'm gonna get you." We crush ourselves instead against God's laws. God has created a universe in which there are natural laws. There are also moral and spiritual laws. And when we violate them, we feel the repercussions of our actions. For example, suppose I drink too much and become intoxicated and then, get in my automobile and drive down the highway at some breakneck speed without control because I am drunk. Whether I want to or not, the laws of motion and stability will be enforced. If I run into a tree, whether I want to or not, my car will crash, and I may be hurt or killed. Or because of my high speed, I may kill other people.

God doesn't will that, but God permits it. God gives us freedom to do God's will or to violate it. God gives me the freedom to abuse my body or to make it stronger. God gives me the freedom to try to learn to do good or to do evil. God gives me the freedom to try to live a moral life or to live an immoral life. God does not force me to conform. When I violate the moral and spiritual laws that are built into the universe, into my life, and into relationships, I often can get hurt. Or I may hurt other people.

Harry Emerson Fosdick said that when he was a young boy his father left the house one Saturday morning and turned to his mother and said, "Tell Harry that he can cut the grass today, if he feels like it." Then he took a few steps and thought for a moment and said, "Tell him that he had better feel like it." When we disobey God, we harm ourselves. God gives us freedom to live in the world. God is not going to confront us with some giant flyswatter to smack us when we sin. But we hurt ourselves as we break the moral and spiritual laws in the universe.

The Seriousness of Sin

Though we may receive forgiveness, and hopefully we will, that does not remove all the consequences that may have resulted from some sinful act. When the prodigal son came home, he was forgiven. But his forgiveness would not undo some problem he may have created in the far country. If he had become involved with some young woman and she became pregnant, his forgiveness would not undo that act. Or if he had engaged in some fight, and he lost a hand, he could receive forgiveness from his father, but his hand would not be restored. God forgives us, but sometimes the consequences of our sinfulness may go on for a long time.

If sin is not considered serious business, we make a mockery of the cross. Whatever else we may want to say about the cross, the cross stands in the center of the universe as the great symbol of God taking sin seriously. We will have to decide whether we will make our own atonement by our own efforts, or whether we will accept God's atonement in Christ. The cross stands as God's love that reaches from eternity into time to touch your life and mine and offers us forgiveness for sin and a new beginning. Forgiveness is serious business and so is sinfulness. But God's love is a great love.

George Buttrick wrote about an experience in the days of the California gold rush. Two sailors were rowing an officer from the mainland of San Francisco to their ship anchored in the bay. The sailors decided that they wanted to be free to see if they could share in the gold rush. So they threw the officer overboard and rowed off to join the search for gold. They were captured and brought back to the ship, court-martialed, and sentenced to be hanged.

A gallows was built on the main deck of the ship to hang the young men. But before they hanged their captors, they decided they would have a service of communion. They went into town and borrowed communion cups, plates, bread, and wine. They invited everyone on the ship to share in the communion service, including the two young murderers whom they were going to hang. There with a gallows before them, they communed about a gallows that had taken place in the past. Remember, the cross was an ancient means of putting people to death. Dr. Buttrick said he wondered if they were engaging in communion because they were aware of the guilt of all and that only a God of holy love can forgive and restore.[7]

There was rich symbolism in that communion service. Maybe they were trying to say that something very unique is commemorated through the event of the death of Christ. Even these two young men, who were about to die, drew strength from the one who died centuries before. Yes, there is a mystery within the death of Christ that has never been totally explained. That is the reason we come again and again to the communion table, because we know that we cannot explain the death of Christ and God's forgiving grace.

The Wonder of Forgiveness

The psalmist reminds us that God's love is sometimes like the compassion of a father who is willing to forgive his children for their sins. "As a father has compassion for his children, so the Lord has compassion for those who fear him" (Ps 103:13). Once I was pastor of a church located a few blocks from a college. We drew a number of university students to our church for worship. I got to know some of them well, and others were total strangers. One day I was called to the hospital to visit a young woman whom I did not know. She had attempted suicide. I went to the hospital and talked with her. She had tried to commit suicide because she was pregnant and didn't know what to do. I talked with her at some length and persuaded her that she had to talk with her parents.

I went back to the church and called a friend of mine who was a pastor in her hometown. I asked him if he knew her parents. He did. In fact, they were members of his church. He told me that he had been playing golf that afternoon with the young woman's father. I asked him, "How will he react?" "I don't know," he said. "He has an explosive temper." "Tell them to come by and talk with me before going to see her," I suggested. They did. Then, they went to the hospital to see their daughter and embraced her and loved her. They knew that it was not the time for condemnation, not the time for rejection, but the time for forgiveness—the time for saying, "Let's begin again." The Scriptures declare to us that, although we are sinners who have all sinned and fallen short of the glory of God, God, nevertheless, reaches out loving arms and draws us unto God's self and says, "I forgive you."

Sin has created a sense of brokenness within us between God, ourselves, and others. Sin has separated us from our true and authentic self. We have been distorted by sin, and sin has distorted our relationship with other people. But God, in gracious forgiveness, offers us an opportunity to build a new bridge, to restore our broken relationship, to help in the restoration of our relationships with others, and to help pull our broken self together. The word salvation means wholeness or fullness. God brings us back together as the authentic persons we were created to be. God's redemption restores us with the quality of life we were created to have. God reveals to us what we can be through the power of that redeeming love.

George Bernard Shaw once stated, in his caustic way, "Forgiveness is nonsense. Everybody must pay his own debt. Forgiveness is a beggar's refuge." But not so. Forgiveness offers us new hope, new opportunity, new beginnings—not a deadend street. When we think that we can't get beyond what we have done, or we are trapped by past mistakes, God offers us opportunities to find fresh beginnings and the strength to continue.

A Higher Standard

Unlike persons to whom the Epistle of John was written, we do not want to set ourselves as the standard for morality. John wrote, "If we say that we have not sinned, we make him [God] a liar, and his word is not in us" (1 John 1:10). To say, "I will be the judge of what is right and what is wrong," is very dangerous. That is partially what is wrong in our society today. We have allowed movies, television, and magazines to determine our standard of morality. And that standard has fallen to the lowest level. Our society has been pervaded with immorality. But that still does not make it right. Just because some say it's ok to cheat, or some say it's ok to steal, or some say it's ok to murder, that does not make it right. If all of society begins to follow the direction of the lowest level of morality, then we will have chaos. Our society will break down, and life will have no meaning.

A higher standard, however, has come into the world and provides guidance for our lives. Now we judge life not by our personal standards, but by the morality of Jesus Christ. I think the Swiss theologian, Karl Barth, was correct when he said that we begin measuring our life not by ourselves but by Christ. When we measure ourselves by Jesus Christ and his standards, then we begin to see how far short we have fallen. The same one by whom we measure our lives is the very one by whom we experience authentic life. Through his righteousness and love, we find forgiveness and grace, and we are able to go on. He has lifted before us the standard on how we should live. He has forgiven us when we have fallen short, but he continuously gives us the strength and courage to follow him.

In France a number of years ago, a group of blind children were taken on a tour of a famous museum. Some of them were led over to a statue called "The Gladiator." Some observers noticed a young boy with short pants standing near the statue. His thin legs were sticking out beneath his short pants, and it was obvious he had a very scrawny body. He reached up, though he could not see, and felt the torso of that massive gladiator. He put his hands around the huge muscles in the statue's body. He felt the huge muscles in his legs. Then that tiny lad straightened up his own body and flexed his muscles. Now, he will never realize the muscular greatness of that figure, but it became a higher goal for him in that moment.

Christ becomes for us the higher model, the clearest example, the highest goal, and the authentic life. Christ has told us: "Love your enemies." "Do unto others as you would have them do unto you." Love becomes the standard that pervades our total life. Although we fall far short, Christ is the standard for our lives.

The psalmist exclaims in Psalm 103:2-5 that we might experience the forgiveness of God in a pit of perdition where we feel we have encountered complete ruin or irreparable loss. Or we may meet God's forgiveness in the depths of death itself. God comes to us and liberates us from our sin. God lifts us up to face life in a new way. Our sins are removed by God "as far as the east is from the west" (v. 12). When God's mercy and forgiveness have had opportunity to work in our lives, our sins are distanced from us.

To Begin Again

Ruel Howe, in a book entitled *The Creative Years*, tells about a young woman who was on the verge of marrying a fine young man.[8] Everybody thought that she was about to begin some delightful and happy years. But a few days before she was to be married, she had a breakdown and was taken to a hospital. No one seemed to be able to do anything with her in the hospital. She simply lay on her bed.

One day an artist, who had been commissioned to paint a portrait for the hospital, heard of this young woman and asked if he might go in and see her. He walked into her room with a lump of clay in his hands and sat down near her bed. Without saying a word, he molded the clay in his fingers. Later he asked the hospital administration if he could visit the young woman again. They felt his visits could be helpful, so he made arrangements to go by her room frequently. For several days he visited her, and no conversation passed between them. He just sat near her, molding his piece of clay. One day she reached over and touched his clay, then quickly drew her hand back.

After several more visits, she reached over and took a piece of the clay in her hand and began to mold and shape it. Then she stopped and threw it against the wall as hard as she could. The artist walked over and picked up the clay and came back smiling and said, "That's ok. Sometimes I feel like doing that to the clay as well. I'm not always satisfied with what I have made either." Slowly she began to talk to him. Soon she took the clay in her hands and began to mold and shape it. From that time on, healing began to come into her life.

During her high school years she had been the head of her class. She had gone to college and graduated as valedictorian. She had been the May Queen and achieved great success. She had always done everything her parents had wanted her to do. She wanted to please them. When she realized that she was getting married, and that she had another person whom she had to please, she didn't know if she could do it. So, she collapsed. The clay symbolized the opportunity to take her life into her own hands and to begin to reshape it.

Our lives can sometimes be twisted, distorted, and broken. But, like clay, they are placed in the hands of the eternal God who is at work in our own lives. Through God's loving, forgiving presence, God takes our life—which may be misshapen, distorted, twisted, broken, or annihilated—and reshapes it into what we were created to be: full, authentic persons. Sin is serious business, but the marvelous good news this day and every day is that in Christ we have found forgiveness and we can begin anew. Let us go on with the journey.

Notes

[1]William S. Stafford, *Disordered Loves: Healing the Seven Deadly Sins* (Cambridge MA: Cowley Publications, 1994) 2.

[2]Walter Rauschenbusch, *A Theology for the Social Gospel* (New York: Macmillan, 1917) 48.

[3]Harvey Cox, *Religion in the Secular City* (New York: Simon & Schuster, 1984) 268.

[4]Harry Stack Sullivan, *The Interpersonal Theory of Psychiatry* (New York: W. W. Norton & Co., 1953) 164.

[5]Paul Tillich, *The Shaking of the Foundations* (New York: Charles Scribner's Sons, 1948) 153-55.

[6]Wolfhart Pannenberg, *The Apostle's Creed in the Light of Today's Questions* (Philadelphia: Westminster Press, 1972) 162-63.

[7]George A. Buttrick, *God, Pain, and Evil* (Nashville: Abingdon Press, 1966) 82-83.

[8]Reuel L. Howe, *The Creative Years* (Greenwich CT: Seabury Press, 1959) 44-48.

Burdens

And what about your prayers, I asked her. Were they left unanswered? You faced a situation that could easily have broken your spirit, a situation that could have left you a bitter, withdrawn woman, jealous of the intact families around you, incapable of responding to the promise of being alive. Somehow that did not happen. Somehow you found the strength not to let yourself be broken. You found the resiliency to go on living and caring about things. Like Jacob in the Bible, like every one of us at one time or another, you faced a scary situation, prayed for help, and found out that you were a lot stronger, and a lot better able to handle it, than you ever would have thought you were. In your desperation, you opened your heart in prayer, and what happened? You didn't get a miracle to avert a tragedy. But you discovered people around you, and God beside you, and strength within you to help you survive the tragedy. I offer that as an example of a prayer being answered.

Harold S. Kushner
When Bad Things Happen to Good People[1]

The problem, it seems to me, is not that suffering and pain exist in the world and that we feel them. The real problem is that suffering seems so random and so meaningless, crushing people as often as it ennobles them, falling upon the undeserving and deserving alike.

William H. Willimon
Sighing for Eden
Sin, Evil, & the Christian Faith[2]

As I meet people each day, I am aware that many have heavy burdens. Some of these burdens are visible but many are invisible. If those in our community who bear burdens marched down Main Street, the clanking of heels would be so loud that we could hardly stand it. Almost everyone bears some kind of burden.

I know a young son who has just put his father in a nursing home. It's hard for him to leave his father there. A daughter has recently taken her mother into her home. She wonders now if she will have enough time for her mother and her own family. The words echoed in the woman's head as she left the doctor's office: "I'm sorry, but it's cancer." A college student is lying in a hospital room. The night before he had been thrown from an automobile, and his spine had been severed. He is paralyzed from the neck down. A family has a fourteen-year-old daughter, but her mind has never developed; she has remained an infant all these years. Her parents have cared for her like a baby through these years and have received very little response from her.

A young teenager wants to make the high school basketball team, but he can't quite get the grades. Now he is thinking of cheating. Another high school student wants to be popular, but for some reasons she has not been drawn into her school group, and now she feels there is only one thing she can do. "I'll drink and behave like the rest," she says. "Then maybe I'll be accepted." A fifty-five-year-old man is called in by his boss: "I'm sorry; you are being replaced soon. Pick up your severance pay at the end of the month." Burdens of all kinds weigh heavily upon us.

Some of you have physical burdens. Your eyesight is failing; your hearing is not as good as it once was. Others suffer from the deterioration of various bodily functions. Financial, personal, or family burdens weigh upon others. Most people carry burdens of one kind or another. Is there any word from the Scriptures about a God who cares? Is there any direction or hope?

In Paul's letter to the Galatian church, Paul states that each one is to bear his own burdens, and, secondly, we are to bear one another's burdens (Gal 6:1-5). The psalmist declares that we are to cast our burdens upon the Lord (Ps 55:22). "Now wait just a minute," we are likely to say. "That doesn't sound possible. It all seems so contradictory." But consider for a moment that these three phrases may be seen as the three sides of a triangle. They each may enable us to discover a different dimension of truth regarding our burdens.

Bear One Another's Burdens

Let's begin with the first one Paul mentions. He says that we are to bear one another's burdens and so fulfill the law of Christ (Gal 6:2). But it is not so popular, is it, to help others bear their load? We had much rather take the approach that someone else's problem is none of our business; let them deal with their own load. We have troubles enough of our own. We had rather be like a turtle—pull our head back into our shell, live in our own realm of personal security. Let someone else deal with his or her problems. They are not my concern. But the turtle, we are told by scientists, is a very insensitive creature. We would like to believe that, as we come up the scale of being to humanity, we will find those who are more sensitive to the needs of others.

There are others who take this approach: "Well, as one looks around in the world, it is really only "the survival of the fittest." That's the kind of universe we live in, isn't it?" "If a person is so weak that she can't make it, that is tough stuff," another says. "After all, look at the forest. It is the big trees that survive. The small ones are soon over-shadowed by the larger ones. They can't get enough rain or sun. They can't get enough nourishment from the soil, and so they quickly die. If a wolf is hurt, the other wolves turn on him, destroy him, and then devour him. You don't put a lamb and a lion in the same cage." Our world is merely a survival of the fittest.

Fulfill the Law of Christ

Is this the Christian approach to life? Paul said, "Bear one another's burdens, and in this way you will fulfill the law of Christ." What law? Where is it written that you are supposed to help others? Paul is talking about the reference to the words of Jesus when he declared that the whole law is fulfilled in loving God with all of your heart and loving your neighbor as yourself. The law of Christ tells you to give yourself in service and concern for someone else. It is creative suffering. That's the law of love. The Greek words Paul uses in this passage about bearing one another's burdens convey an image about the cargo on a ship being properly balanced. The cargo had to be distributed on those ancient ships in proper balance and proportion so the ship might sail effectively. When our burden or load is properly distributed, we can handle it more easily because others are helping us bear the load.

I once heard Dr. Roger Omanson, a New Testament scholar and linguist, say that when the Good News Bible was first translated, one of the pen drawings depicting this verse in Galatians was called into question. The drawing showed a group of people walking in a line carrying a load of some kind. In the line were two men, a woman, a small boy, and a little girl. Each was helping in some way to assist the person in front of him or her. But the young girl at the end of the line had no one behind her to help her carry her load. There was so much criticism about the figure of the girl bearing her load by herself that in the next edition of the New Testament it showed a hand reaching out from behind her from a person who obviously continued the line of figures as he gave her support with her burden. Each person had someone helping him or her bear the load. This helps capture something of Paul's image of our responsibility to help bear the load of one another as we go through life.

Live in the Present

A remarkable thing happens when we reach out to help someone else. It enables us to live in the present. Too many people remember or focus only on the good they did for someone in the past, or they keep talking about what they want to do for someone in the future, but they really do not do much for other people in the present moment. Do you remember the story about the children of Israel when they were in the wilderness? They received manna from God to eat, but God told them that they were to gather only enough for each day, because they could not hoard it for tomorrow. Each day they had to gather a fresh supply. That can serve as a reminder to us about our own way of living. We cannot live simply on what we have done in the past. Whatever good or service we may have done in the past does not mean that more is not needed today. We are challenged to keep on doing good today and in the tomorrows ahead of us.

You remember the story about the man who went to a friend to borrow some money. His friend said, "I can't do any more for you." "But you have never done anything for me," the borrower exclaimed. "What do you mean I have never done anything for you?" his friend responded. "I saved you from drowning once. I have lent you thousands of dollars in the past." "That's right," the borrower replied, "but what have you done for me lately?" There is some truth in that response. It is not enough to speak about what we have done in the past, but the way we help our fellow human beings bear their burdens today keeps our life focusing on present needs and fills it with meaning and richness.

Strengthen Your Life

When you help others in their struggles, it also strengthens your own life. When you reach out to help someone else who is struggling with their load, you discover that you are fortified and strengthened yourself as you help them. A muscle is strengthened by exercise. If you don't use certain muscles, they become weak and flabby, but the more you use them, the stronger they become. The more you exercise your "muscle of helpfulness " by reaching out to someone in need, the stronger your own gift of concern and caring will become through its use.

I have discovered in churches where I have pastored that when people are crushed down by tragedy or heavy burdens, it is helpful to send a person who has had a similar problem to minister to them. If these persons have experienced the death of a child, an accident, a prolonged illness, or some other kind of burden and they have found strength from Christ and the church, they can go to other individuals who are experiencing similar problems and help undergird them and bear their load. When they have been strengthened, they can help strengthen others. Those who have lost a child by death, have difficulty in hearing, or bear some other burden, can speak to those with similar problems and say, "I know your ache; I sense your need; I have been there; I understand." And you know they do.

One day I was working in my yard trying to gather up a deluge of branches and sticks that had blown down from the trees after fifty-mile-an-hour winds cut through them. As I picked up the sticks to put them in trash bags, it wasn't hard to break a small bundle of them. But it really was amazing how difficult it became when the pile got larger. It was almost impossible to break them when they were grouped together. As I gathered up those sticks, I thought about life's burdens. When we try to carry our burdens by ourselves, they can crush us. They seem too much for us. But when we draw on the strength of fellow Christians and our church community to undergird us and support us, we find a source of strength that enables us to face difficulties we never thought we could meet.

Fellow Christians strengthen and undergird us as we struggle with our load of pain and grief. With the assistance of others, we are made stronger and, as we are strengthened by them, we in turn reach out to minister to others. It would be impossible for any one or two people to visit all the lonely, shut-in, ill, or grieving church members, but as a community, you can help bear the load. Not only do you strengthen others by your help, but you are stronger yourself because of this ministry of concern.

Overcome Self-Centeredness

When you help others with their burdens, you also find that it helps you overcome your self-centeredness. It gets your mind off yourself. There are some people who play what I call the "Oh pity me" or "Ain't it awful?" games all the time. "Nobody could have it as bad as I have it," they state. They sit at home and moan and groan about their problems, looking inwardly all the time and unable to face themselves and their burdens and go on.

I know a woman who played these evasive games until finally she was pulled out of her self-centeredness by becoming involved in helping other people who had needs greater than her own. She began to visit others in their home or in the hospital. She baked pies or cakes and took them to the homes of people who were sick or grieving. As she tried to help them, an astounding thing happened. She forgot all about her own problems because she was so busy helping others with their needs.

Bear one another's burdens and so fulfill the law of Christ. We are challenged to move out of our self-centeredness and reach out to minister to others. This is the law of Christ; it is the law of service, the law of concern, and the law of grace.

Bear Your Own Burden

Paul also notes that each one is to bear his or her own burden (Gal 6:5). There are some loads in life that no one else can bear for you. No one else can be born for you, and no one else is going to die for you. There are some things in life that you must bear isolated and alone. You are responsible for your own sin. There is a sense of sinfulness that is uniquely your own. Each of us is a sinner, and that is a burden each bears.

A woman called her minister one day and told him that she needed to talk with him. The woman told the minister about a sordid love affair she had had. He listened sympathetically to her as she tried to find some way to have forgiveness for what she had done. He reminded her about God's grace and forgiveness. "Great is your sinfulness," he said, "but great is God's forgiveness." She was able to find forgiveness that day and begin anew. Our burden of sin can find release in the power of God's grace.

Guilt

Some of you are burdened with guilt over acts you have done in the past or things you have not done, for something you have said, or not said. Guilt crushes you down to the ground with its heavy load.

Several years ago a naturalist found a large eagle with an animal trap on its leg. This huge eagle had gotten caught by a trap that was set to catch small animals. By the strength of its powerful wings and body, the eagle was able to break the trap loose from the ground and fly off with it. After a while the trap became so heavy that the eagle could not fly with it, and the load pulled the bird down to the ground. The eagle was found dead along the seashore.

Some of you carry a heavy load of guilt and have never received release from it. You have not heard God's words of grace: "You are acceptable, and you are forgiven; begin anew." You can receive those words now and experience release.

Grief

Others of you find that your own individual burden is grief. As the prophet Jeremiah exclaimed, "This is my grief, and I must bear it." There are some aspects about personal grief that no one else can bear for you, not even a close friend or a minister. No one else can bear your grief totally for you. A part of grief is your own very personal inner struggle; it is your own load, and you know you must shoulder it. You search now for ways you can handle it.

Others are burdened with problems of arthritis, failing eyesight, deafness, heart trouble, a lung condition, or other kinds of physical ailments. Some have financial or other kinds of burdens. At times, these burdens seem too heavy, and you feel that they will be too much for you to bear. How will you respond to your personal burden? Will you let your burden make you bitter toward life? Or will you be able to meet it with a positive perspective?

Your Attitude

Lord Byron, the English poet, and his friend, Sir Walter Scott, the English writer, were both lame. But Byron always viewed his lameness with great bitterness and complained and brooded about it constantly. Scott never mentioned his disability to anyone. One day Lord Byron wrote a letter to the famous English writer and observed: "Ah Scott, I would give all my fame to have your happiness." What was the difference in these two men? The attitude they took toward their burden made the difference.

A medical doctor lost his nine-year-old daughter to leukemia. What did he do? Did he sulk and become bitter? No! After the tragic death of his daughter, he determined he would do everything he could to help young children in our nation. He established children's homes across this country to provide a home for children who had no place to live. Rather than becoming bitter, he directed his energies toward doing something positive to help others who had burdens. Your attitude toward the burdens you bear can determine your perspective. You cannot always control what happens to you. The circumstances in which you find yourself may be beyond your control or anyone else's, but the attitude you take toward these circumstances can make all the difference in how you meet whatever burdens you have to bear.

When Corrie ten Boom and her Dutch family were imprisoned in a German concentration camp by the Nazis in the Second World War, one of the guards said to her, "The only way you can survive in this place is by hating." "Hate," she responded, "can put you in a prison worse than this." Bitterness can make your life miserable. Hatred can make your life morbid. Your attitude may not change the conditions in which you find yourself, but it can affect the way you adjust to them.

George Frideric Handel had a paralytic stroke at age fifty-six and was living in poverty when he wrote his magnificent "Hallelujah Chorus." Helen Keller, who was blind and deaf, wrote, "I thank God for my handicap because through it I found myself, my work, and God." In 1812, a young man was working in his father's harness shop. An accident caused some of the tools to fly into his face and put out his eyes. Several years later, Braille invented a system so blind people could read with their fingers. His blindness led to a whole new way of seeing for thousands of other blind people around the world.

R. T. Van was at one time president of Meredith College in Raleigh, North Carolina. When he was a young man, he lost both arms in an accident. Later a student said to him, "Dr. Van, just think what you could have done if you had both of your arms." "If I had not lost my arms," Dr. Van responded, "I might still be on the farm in North Carolina. It was because of my loss that I determined to do something with myself which otherwise might not have happened." His attitude made the difference.

When I was a pastor in Virginia, I received word about the death of a young man named David Ken Miller in Johnson City, Tennessee. David Miller had had polio when he was six-years-old and was completely paralyzed. He could not care for himself in any way. He even had to be put in a brace to sit in a wheelchair. His father was robbed and murdered when David was only nine years old. His mother became the sole support for the family. With her help, David finished Lamar High School and then went to East Tennessee State University and graduated magna cum laude. The university students used to take turns rolling his wheelchair across campus to classes. He received national publicity when he was in a college friend's wedding and an iron lung was sought for him to sleep in on the night before the wedding. He slept in an iron lung most of his life.

David was active in community and civic affairs. He taught teenagers in a local Baptist church. He was employed as a fourth-grade teacher. The students were devoted to him, and the highest honor of the day was to be selected to feed Mr. Miller at lunch time. The night before he died, he had been elected chairman of the Uneka Committee, a committee for the improvement of life for the physically handicapped in the city where he lived. The Easter Seal Society gave him its highest national honor—the Gallantry Award. He also received posthumously the Governor's Citation for Achievement. This young man was completely paralyzed—unable to use his legs, arms, or body, but he used his mind and all of the gifts he had to their fullest. His attitude made the difference in how he chose to live.

Everyone has some burden at one time or another. You will discover your burden, and you will have to bear it. You may not be able to control what happens to you, but you can determine how you will respond to what happens. The word for burden in the passage from Galatians is the word for a soldier's load or pack. All of us have a certain load we are responsible for carrying. Like soldiers, we take the load on our shoulders and move on under its weight.

Cast Your Burden on the Lord

Although we bear one another's burdens and each one must bear his or her burden, ultimately, we can cast our burdens upon the Lord. To cast our burden upon the Lord is not a stoic approach that says "grit your teeth and bear it." To cast your burden upon the Lord is to draw upon the power that can sustain you beyond your own strength or the efforts of others. It is to be able to say with Corrie ten Boom in the midst of a terrible ordeal in a German concentration camp, "There is no pit so deep that God is not deeper still." God is present with you to help bear the load of pain, suffering, ache, or sorrow.

But note carefully. It does not mean that you lose all of your burdens by casting them on God. Paul prayed that his thorn in the flesh might be removed, but it was not. Jesus prayed in Gethsemane, "Oh, Lord God, let this cup of suffering pass," but it did not. You may pray for your burden to be removed. But . . . Your hearing may not be restored. Your eyesight may not get better. You may not be free of your cancer. Whatever your burden is, it may not be completely lifted, but the biblical promise is that you can still trust God. Nothing can ultimately separate you from God (Rom 8:35-39).

God has not promised that you will never have problems or difficulties, but God has promised to be with you in the midst of them. Jesus said, "Take my yoke upon you. . . . My burden is light" (Matt 11:29, 30). Christ undergirds you with his power, sustains you with his grace, and gives you the assurance that no matter what you may have to bear, you do not bear it individually or in isolation, or rely merely on the strength of others. Underneath is the power and presence of God. God is always there to sustain you.

Several years ago I had the privilege of eating a meal with Merrill Womack, the famous religious singer. On Thanksgiving Day in 1961, his private plane crashed and burned. His face was burned so badly that he was totally disfigured. Over the years, he has had more than seventy skin graft operations on his face. When you first meet him, you might experience some discomfort and unpleasantness because of his appearance. But, when he stands up to sing, you forget his face. He has a magnificent voice that has been praised all over this country for its beauty and quality.

After his accident, Merrill said that he had reached the point of no return in his life. He didn't know if he could go on. But down in the darkest valley he found the presence of Christ, and he has returned. A movie entitled *He Restoreth My Soul* has been made about his life and how he was sustained by the presence of God in the midst of the darkest moment of his life. Here is one who can exclaim that God was still with him in the worst kinds of circumstances and continues to bear him up in the midst of his tragedy. He has not been forsaken by God.

Merrill Womack continues through his singing to give testimony to the sustaining presence and power of God.

Remember, there are some burdens you must bear by yourself. Don't forget to continue to help others as they struggle with their load, but always remember that underneath you as you struggle with your burdens is the God who will sustain you.

Phillips Brooks, the noted Boston preacher, expressed the assurance of God's presence in these lines:

Our Burden Bearer

The little sharp vexations
And the briars that catch and fret,
why not take all to the Helper
Who has never failed us yet?
Tell Him about the heartache,
And tell Him the longings, too;
Tell Him the baffled purpose
When we scarce know what to do.
Then, leaving all our weakness
With One divinely strong,
Forget that we bore the burden,
And carry away the song.

Notes

[1]Harold S. Kushner, *When Bad Things Happen to Good People* (New York: Schockon Books, 1981) 130-31.
[2]William H. Willimon, *Sighing for Eden: Sin, Evil, & the Christian Faith* (Nashville: Abingdon Press, 1985) 164.

Suffering

The most profound dimension that could be opened to the victim is that in the midst of the enigma of suffering, he or she could encounter the Numinous One. Some may have glimpsed a Some one who faintly beckoned to them from within their suffering. One might envision this One as inviting them to imagine a hidden purpose and significance for living that they could not rationally fashion.

Daniel Liderbach
Why Do We Suffer?[1]

Cancer has pushed my reset button. I can't live for others anymore. I don't mean I want to become selfish. There's a great difference between being self-centered and being centered in one's self. I have to be satisfied with me and my life, whether or not anyone else is.

Day by day now, I feel a little more comfortable with walking the lonesome valley by myself. I think that's a good sign. It means I'm beginning to understand that my justification for living is just that I'm here. My meaning comes from inside. All that I need for facing life, yes, and for facing death, God has already put into my life.

John Robert McFarland
Now That I Have Cancer I Am Whole[2]

The question was on everyone's lips. Why? Why did it happen? I was a graduate student at Emory University in Atlanta, Georgia. Early Sunday morning on June 4, 1962, an Air France jet crashed and burned upon takeoff near Paris. All of the 132 passengers aboard were killed except the two stewardesses who were thrown to safety when the tail section of the plane broke off. Killed in this flaming crash were many of the civic and cultural leaders of Atlanta. "Why does God allow such things to happen?" people asked. Quick came the response: "It was the will of God. Accept it." But was it?

Two missionary couples in China discovered that their children had diphtheria. They both prayed to God that their children might be spared. One of the children died; the other lived. Some said to the missionary couple, "It is the will of God. Accept it." But was it?

Some had sons or husbands go off to war and prayed to God that they might return safely. Some have and some have not. People have often said, "Accept it. It is the will of God." But is it?

A university professor was hit by a passing car as he was crossing the street and was hospitalized. The first time he had an opportunity to lecture at school, he stood before the students and said, "I no longer believe in God, because if there were a God who existed, God should have whispered in my ear and warned me of that approaching car so I would not have been hurt. I do not believe in God."

Several years ago in Nelson County, Virginia, part of a mountain-side slid away and killed hundreds of people in that community. I sat in a small country church and participated in a funeral service with five caskets in front of me. They were all from one family. Some said that this suffering was the will of God, to accept it. But was it?

Leslie Weatherhead, the noted London preacher, was sitting in India on a veranda talking to a father who was grieving over the death of his only son in the dread cholera epidemic. The father looked up at the minister and said, "Well, Padre, it is the will of God. That's all there is to it. It is the will of God."

His only daughter lay sleeping under a mosquito net at the other side of the veranda. Dr. Weatherhead, knew the man rather well, and so he asked him:

> Supposing someone crept up the steps onto the veranda tonight, while you all slept, and deliberately put a wad of cotton soaked in cholera germ over your little girl's mouth as she lay in that cot there on the veranda. What would you think about that?

The father quickly snapped back:

> My God, what would I think about that?. . . If he attempted it, and I caught him, I would kill him with as little compunction as I would a snake and throw him over the veranda. What do you mean by suggesting such a thing?

Weatherhead continued:

> But John, isn't that just what you have accused God of doing when you said it was His will? Call your little boy's death the result of

mass ignorance, call it mass folly, call it mass sin, if you like, call it bad drains or communal carelessness, but don't call it the will of God. Surely we cannot identify as the will of God something for which a man would be locked up in jail or put in a criminal lunatic asylum.[3]

Too often we call some events the will of God that should never be credited that way. I want to attempt to address the problem of evil, suffering, tragedy, and pain. I shall not give these questions some glib or simple answer, because I feel there is none. Phillips Brooks once remarked that if someone should tell him that he could explain the mystery of evil and suffering, he would close his ears to that offer. Rather than telling you I have all of the answers to the questions of suffering and evil, I would like to offer some pathways that might lead us in the right direction through the darkness.

An Adequate Concept of God

When we talk about evil, suffering, pain, and death, we have to begin with an adequate or valid concept of God. Too often our concept of God is almost demonic. God is depicted as though God were a fiend who demands a pound of flesh. God is often depicted as revengeful, vindictive, implacable, uncaring, and unmerciful. The kind of God who would deliberately send suffering, pain, cancer, and heart attacks upon us could be seen only as an enemy. We would put a person in jail for the kind of things we often attribute so quickly and easily to God.

How do you see God? Does God see a young woman in good health, who loves to swim and play tennis, and decide deliberately to send polio into her life? Does God select a young man who enjoys playing football, basketball, and other sports and send him cancer so he loses his leg? Would you say that kind of God was a God of love or a God who was a fiend? To assume that God's will is to send suffering, broken bodies, cancer, accidents, and pain is to declare that God is demonic. We need to be very careful that we do not blame God for sending all suffering and pain upon us as though it were God's intent. To say that someone wills something is to indicate that he or she wants it to happen. To say that God wills suffering means that God wants it to come into our lives. Think what kind of image of God that portrays.

In an H. G. Wells novel, Mr. Britling asserts, "Why, if I thought there was a God who looked down on battles and death and all the horrors of war, able to prevent these things. . . I would spit into his empty face." This type of God should be cursed. What kind of God would create a world and, then, deliberately send suffering and pain upon those children? Only a fiend would do that. When we picture God in this way, we have a very distorted concept of God's nature. Surely we cannot maintain as a Christian concept that God willfully sends evil, calamity, disease, pain, and suffering upon us.

We need an adequate concept of God that we see in Jesus Christ. The Scriptures do not depict a God who is demonic, hateful, and mean. In Jesus Christ, God has been revealed as a God of love and grace. God's nature is redemptive love. From Jesus, we have learned that God is like a father who cares for His children. Jesus taught us that not a sparrow falls to the ground without the knowledge of God and that the hairs of our head are all numbered. The New Testament depicts God, not as a God of vengeance and hate, but of love and grace. We understand more clearly what God is like by beginning with the image of God we have seen in Jesus Christ. Love is the basic force we see there. The cross on Calvary's hill is evidence of the cross of love in the heart of God. If we are to find any direction, we begin with an adequate concept of God.

An Adequate Concept of the Universe

When we talk about evil, suffering, pain, and death, we also need an adequate concept of the universe. In a previous chapter I spoke about sin. Unfortunately, in our English language we have only one word to describe evil. In German there are two different words for evil, one for human sin and another for natural evil. Unfortunately, in English we cannot separate the two clearly, because we have only one word to describe both moral and natural evil. There is no question that you and I sin. Sin is our personal rebellion against God, others, and ourselves. But there is also natural evil in our universe. This evil does not always come about through our own choice or the deeds of human kind; it is a result of the natural operation of the universe itself. An adequate concept of the law-abiding nature of the universe has been helpful to me in understanding the problem of suffering and evil.

God has created our universe so that it is a law abiding realm. Think of the chaotic state of the world if there were no laws in the universe on which we could depend. If the natural realm had no dependable laws, then we could not know from one moment to the next whether the chair we are sitting in would hold us up or suddenly change to something else. How could we have a house to live in if we did not know whether the ceiling and floor would remain in their proper places? If your car could suddenly become a pumpkin without warning, think what kind of mass confusion would exist in the world. If there were nothing stable or dependable within the universe, we would live in a world of chaos and horror. Dr. John Whale, an English theologian, expressed it this way:

> If water might suddenly freeze in midsummer, if the specific gravity of lead might at any time become that of thistledown, if pigs might fly, if the Houses of Parliament turn into green-cheese—man's life would become a nightmare.[4]

God did not make us to be robots; God created us with free will. You and I, and all humanity, have to learn to live in cooperation with the laws of the universe. God has created laws that are operating in the world, and we have to learn how these laws function and how to live in accordance with these laws. When my children were small and I taught them not to place their hands on a red hot burner on a stove, I don't think I was going against the will of God. When I taught them not to play with matches, I was not going against the will of God. When I taught them not to play with razor blades and not to run out in the street in front of a car, I was not going against the will of God. I was teaching them to learn to live in cooperation with the dependable laws of the universe. If I climb to the top of a tall building and jump off, I can't decide halfway down that I don't want to jump. The law of gravity will be enforced. If we are trying to teach our children not to get burned, hurt, cut, or killed, why do we say that it is the will of God when one of the very things we were teaching them to avoid happens? Call it an accident or the deliberate abuse of the laws of the universe, but do not call it the will of God.

Living with the Laws of the Universe

We live in a universe where God has set natural laws in operation, and, as a part of this universe, we have to learn to live in accordance with them. Sometimes, when the natural laws of the universe are in operation, devastation may occur to a city or people who are in the path of a tornado, an earthquake, or a hurricane, but that doesn't mean that God has sent it. These natural forces are working in cooperation with the laws that God has established within the created world. God expects us to learn how to live in the universe. God has given us free will and does not deny us our right to express it, even when God knows that through our use of it, we might sometimes get hurt.

But hear this word also from the Scriptures: When God created the universe, he looked upon his creation and said it was "good" (Gen 1:31). God did not say that it was perfect, final, nor complete. In our understanding of the orderly nature of the universe, let us be aware that God is not remote and removed from God's creation but is still actively involved in the creative process. God did not set our world spinning and then remove God's self from its operation. God is still guiding creation toward its ultimate goal. In the same epistle to the Roman Church, Paul declared that "the creation itself will be set free from its bondage to decay and will obtain the freedom of the glory of the children of God" (Rom 8:21). The universe itself is still groaning in travail and moving toward fulfillment. The universe is moving toward redemption. As persons who are still in the process of being made whole, all of God's universe is proceeding toward wholeness and redemption.

Why insects, disease, and germs are allowed in the creation seems a mystery to us. When a mosquito is biting my arm or leg, I do not know what its beneficial effect is. But the mosquito has some useful function in creation other than providing food for some creatures. I don't know what these functions are, but obviously it has some. Leslie Weatherhead has suggested that in some ways, unknown to us, in the scheme of the universe, these creatures of destruction may serve or have served some useful function. Few of us, he notes, are aware that the pesky wasps in nine out of ten of its activities are helpful. From late spring to early autumn, they seek out and destroy vast numbers of caterpillars and grubs that, if left unchecked, would destroy crops, vegetables, orchards, and trees.[5]

I do not know why viruses, diphtheria, TB, AIDS, or cancer exist. You and I may not know what is the ultimate purpose of these kinds of things or if they have any beneficial purpose, but, when we combat them, we are certainly not acting in opposition to the will of God. When doctors or scientists battle against disease to find a cure or labor to control insects, they do not oppose the will of God. Although God has created a universe where illness and misfortune are possible, God is good and does not deliberately send anything to hurt us or harm us.

The Power of God

A third issue focuses on the power of God. If God is good, and if God is all-powerful, why is there suffering, pain, and evil in the world? Why do they exist? If God is omnipotent, or all-powerful, why, then, does God not prevent evil? Why does God allow suffering? Why is pain in our world? Why does it exist? Why hasn't God created a world in which there is no possibility of suffering, pain, death, or grief?

In Archibald MacLeish's play *J.B.*, the question is raised: "If God is God, He is not good. If God is good, He is not God."[6] If God is a good God, why does God not use that divine power to free us from all the evil in the world? If God lacks the power to help, is God really omnipotent? Jesus Christ has revealed to us that God is good. But this does not imply that a "good" God has not set some "limits" upon that divine power. God did not spare Jesus from suffering, pain, and death. God is "limited" by the freedom given to creation to make choices. God has "limited" God's self to a degree by human freedom and natural laws. God has created the world in such a way that there is no possibility of good without the possibility of evil. There is no possibility of positive behavior without the possibility of negative behavior. There is no possibility of being brave without, at the same time, the possibility of being cowardly. There is no possibility of being kind without at the same time the possibility of being unkind.

God has created this kind of world because without freedom, there is no potential for growth. Without freedom, there is no potential for choice. We would only be robots. God does not have us on a string manipulating us through life. We are free, moral agents. God gives us a choice. God has given humans freedom, and God has built freedom into the structure of the universe itself. As the universe is growing and expanding, we have opportunity to grow and expand. God does not want us to sin, but God has created us with the freedom to make choices. And because we choose to sin does not mean that God wants us to sin. God, nevertheless, permits it. God has given us freedom. If we did not have the possibility of sinning, we would not really have free will. But freedom is an essential element in the world God designed.

The Possibility of Growth

I do not think for a moment that God wants suffering and pain for us. God has permitted them because without them, growth is not possible. If I could raise a gun, point it at you, and pull the trigger, and, then, in midair the bullet would suddenly become water, killing would not exist. Or, if I could walk into a bank and rob it of a million dollars, and then, as soon as I left, a million dollars would fill the vacuum, robbery would have no meaning. Or, if I could steal your automobile and as soon as I drove off, another automobile would take its place, stealing would be a meaningless word. If I raised a knife to stab you, and it turned into a piece of paper, natural laws would not be reliable.

If this were the kind of universe we lived in, where no one could be harmed or no wrong could ever be done to another, there would be no possibility of morality, virtue, good character, honesty, courage, perseverance, or love. All of these values would not exist without a world where suffering, sin, injustice, and evil are realities. How could there be moral or immoral qualities or good or evil where there is no such thing as suffering, danger, uncertainty, and challenge? If we have no choice and our actions are already decided, we are not authentic persons but pawns on a chess board who are totally controlled by another. God has given us freedom of choice as we live in the universe God created. Through our choices we have opportunity to grow and mature.

In the book of Isaiah, the author declares that God is the source of good and ultimately the source of evil, because God has created the possibility of both. "I am the Lord, there is no other; I make the light, I create darkness, author alike of prosperity and trouble" (Isa 45:7 NEB). God does not deliberately send evil upon us, but God has created the kind of universe where both good and evil are realities. God is the author of all things, because God has created the possibility of either existing.

Are Christians Exempt?

Some have raised the question: "Does God spare Christians from suffering and pain?" There are some who tell us that if we will pray hard enough, have enough faith, and think positive thoughts, God will protect us from all suffering, pain, and evil. Sometimes much harm has been done by that approach. My experience has taught me how untrue this is. I have sat by sick beds of dedicated Christians who have suffered great agony and pain. I have walked to the cemetery with families of some of the finest Christian men, women, and young people I have ever known. Some of the most faithful saints have suffered years of intense pain and trouble. But God has not promised us that because we are Christians we will be spared all suffering and pain. God has not offered us a magic way of escape. God's own Son was not spared suffering and death. As Dorothy Soelle said,

> Living like Christ will not mean reward, social recognition and an assured income, but difficulties, discrimination, solitude, anxiety. The message of Jesus is that the more you grow in love, the more vulnerable you make yourself.[7]

In Luke 21:8-19, Jesus stated that Christians might suffer wars, physical calamities, economic loss, and many other distresses. In the Epistle to the Romans, Paul reminds us that, although Christians are not exempt from suffering, nothing can separate us from God's presence. In the midst of all our suffering, God is present with us. This passage does not mean that everything that happens to us is the will of God, but it does teach us that *in all things* God is working to bring about good. Even in the worst kind of circumstances, God works in our lives to bring good from it. This does not imply that it is good for you to be in pain, but that in or through your pain, God may bring goodness, hope, and new possibilities for growth.

I have known people who have looked up at me from sick beds and asked, "Pastor, why? I have tried to be a good Christian. Why is God doing this to me?" But God did not send sickness upon them. God is, nevertheless, present with them in their difficulty. Nothing in all creation—whether it is pain or suffering, life or death, in the present or future—can separate us from the love of God we have experienced in Jesus Christ.

In Romans 5, Paul acknowledges that Christians often suffer in this life. But he affirms that growth may occur through our suffering, pain, or tragedy. Our troubles—literally pressures such as persecution, sorrow, pain, or unpopularity—may press in upon us from all quarters. These troubles or pressures lead to fortitude or endurance. Fortitude is the spirit that meets head-on and overcomes the trials it encounters. This endurance produces character. Like metal that has been fired, the Christian has been refined in the fire of tribulation. Like sterling silver that has been purged in fire and is now free of alloys, the Christian has passed through the fires of suffering and is now a "sterling" or noble creature because of the difficulties she has faced. Out of all of our suffering and pain, God has brought about the process of our growth and we have become stronger persons because of our sufferings.

God's Grace

God does not remove Christians from suffering but assures us of the divine presence even in the midst of our sufferings. Think of what some have accomplished even under great hardship or suffering. Some of the finest individuals down through history have suffered. John Milton wrote some of his greatest poetic works after he became blind. Beethoven became deaf, but out of his deafness came marvelous music. Although he could not hear it, others rejoiced in its sound. Dostoevski, the Russian novelist, suffered from epilepsy. Louis Pasteur suffered a paralytic stroke at the age of forty-six, but some of his greatest discoveries came after his stroke. Alexander Pope was sickly and deformed in body, but he dominated English literature most of his life. The apostle Paul cried out to God, "O Lord, remove this thorn in my flesh." But God replied, "My grace is sufficient for you."

God does not promise us as Christians that we will be spared all suffering and pain. But God tells us that divine grace will sustain us. The word for grace is an image of one being ushered into the presence of royalty. We are introduced into the presence of God by the sustaining power of the Son. The word grace also contains an image of a ship finding refuge in a harbor. We have a safe harbor or haven from the stresses of life when we are in the grace of Christ. He sustains us. God has not removed all of our troubles, tribulations, suffering, and difficulties, but God is there in the midst of them to sustain us. And we know that, when we are sustained by God, we have a peace that cannot be overwhelmed. God works in all things for good.

An Answerer

The only satisfying answer to the dilemma of pain and suffering, according to Douglas John Hall, "is the answer given to Job—the answer that is no answer but is the presence of an Answerer." He continues with this insight about the presence of God in our suffering:

> It does not matter that the Answerer brings more questions than answers; for the answer is not the words as such but the living Word—the Presence itself. The answer is the permission that is given in this Presence to be what one is, to express the dereliction that belongs to one's age and place, to share all of it with this Other: to *trample!* Faith is the communion of the spirit with this fellow sufferer, this One whose otherness lies in the fact that he will not turn away in the face of one's failure, or in the failure of one's world.[8]

Have you ever heard how a real Persian rug is made? A frame is built to support the rug, and some small boys sit on one side of the rug. The expert designer or artist is on the other side and shouts his instructions to them. The young boys feed the colored thread through the rug as he guides them to the design he has in his mind. Sometimes the designer may walk off for a few minutes, and while he is away one of the young boys may carelessly push some of his thread in the wrong direction or may not follow the pattern exactly. A great artist will not ask the boy to pull out the color and start over, but he weaves the mistake into the overall pattern of the rug so that it blends in with the rest of the pattern. Here is a parable for us.

When suffering and pain come into your life and my life, God does not promise us that we will be spared. But we are assured that God will work in and through this difficulty to blend it into our lives and the lives of our family and community to bring out of it something good and worthwhile. God does not exempt us from suffering and sin, but God is an artist who can bring beauty, wholeness, and good out of agony and wrong. We know that in God's grace we can withstand all things, because God is present with us to uphold us and enable us to meet all circumstances. A valid concept of God and the universe will help us in our struggle with the problem of evil and suffering. Lean heavily on God's grace to sustain you. God is present in all situations, and God will never let you down.

Notes

[1]Daniel Liderbach, *Why Do We Suffer?* (New York: Paulist Press, 1992) 128.
[2]John Robert McFarland, *Now That I Have Cancer I Am Whole* (Kansas City MO: Andrews and McMeel, 1993) 79-80.

[3]Leslie D. Weatherhead, *The Will of God* (New York: Abingdon Press, 1944) 10-11.

[4]John Whale, *The Christian Answer to the Problem of Evil* (London: SCM, 1957) 28.

[5]Leslie D. Weatherhead, *Why Do Men Suffer?* (New York: Abingdon Press, 1936) 66.

[6]Archibald MacLeish, *J. B.* (Boston: Houghton Mifflin, 1958) 14.

[7]Dorothy Soelle, *Thinking about God: An Introduction to Theology* (Philadelphia: Trinity Press, 1990) 133-34.

[8]Douglas John Hall, *God and Human Suffering* (Minneapolis MN: Augsburg, 1986) 118.

Unanswerable Questions

AIDS

We have AIDS. Faced with the present urgency, we as a global community recognize our brokenness and common need for healing and reconciliation. Together as a community we must continue to struggle toward genuine acceptance of and respect for each individual person. To do this, we must overcome prejudice and discrimination. We are not called to be judgmental. We are called to be a healing church. We believe that all people are equal before God. AIDS is a disease that highlights the fragmented nature of our world. It frightens many into a response of isolation, injustice, and abandonment of those in need. Such responses are contrary to the scriptural mandate of reconciliation. AIDS challenges us into a new level of introspection and communication that releases the energy of human hope, courage, and love. The supreme challenge of AIDS is for the church truly to be God's agent of love and reconciliation in the world.

We, the body of Christ, in this moment of history, have AIDS. We have a loving, tender, merciful, and compassionate God who walks with us on our journey.

Letty M. Russell
The Church with AIDS[1]

The AIDS epidemic provides the church of Jesus Christ with an opportunity to express loving compassion. AIDS is a new, different sort of disease. Consequently, dealing with people who have been affected by the disease may well be the greatest challenge our modern-day churches have. Ironically, AIDS may also force many contemporary churches to examine their motives for existence, to rediscover their mission in the world, and to reconnect with the Power to get that mission accomplished.

Jimmy Allen
Burden of a Secret[2]

Weeks had slipped into months as I had talked with this young man. He had come to see me nervously to begin with, but John Smith (not his real name) wanted to know if he could trust me and whether or not he could be confidential with me. After talking with him for some time, he revealed to me that he had AIDS. As the months went by, he went into the hospital. We had numerous conversations while he was in the hospital.

Soon we both knew that he was not going to leave the hospital again. We had spoken about many of his fears before, but on this day he looked up at me and asked, "Pastor, have I committed the unpardonable sin?" This young man joins the ranks of many today in our world who are suffering and dying from AIDS.

The Devastating March

AIDS is no respecter of persons. Young or old, men or women, married or single, children or babies, learned or unlearned, black or white, red or yellow, all, under certain circumstances, can fall victim to the dreaded disease of AIDS. The faces of many have crossed our line of vision, and their images haunt us. Persons from various segments of society have contracted AIDS. The list includes Rock Hudson; Liberace; Ryan White; Arthur Ashe; Kimberly Bengalis; Ali Gertz; an Olympic medal winner; a congressman; a church bishop; Elizabeth Glasser and her daughter, Ariel; Magic Johnson with the HIV infection; the journalist Randy Shilts; and countless artists, poets, writers, musicians, actors, and persons from every walk of life. Perhaps someone from your own family could be added to the list of those who have died from AIDS.

The scourge of AIDS has spread across equatorial Africa, the Caribbean, Central and South America, and into North America. It is now beginning to make its way across Asia and Eastern Europe. The first case of AIDS was reported in our country in 1981. Today AIDS is a worldwide problem. The World Health Organization estimates that 18,000,000 adults and 1,500,000 children are infected with the HIV virus, and by the turn of the century, 30,000,000-40,000,000 people will be infected with HIV.[3] The Centers for Disease Control estimates that 1,000,000 Americans are infected with HIV, a figure that translates to 1 in every 160 men and 1 in every 1,000 women. Through June 1996, 548,102 men, women, and children with AIDS have been reported to CDC; 343,000 have died. AIDS is now the sixth leading cause of premature death in America.[4] On World AIDS Day in December 1996, it was estimated that 6,400,000 people had died with AIDS. This tragedy is compounded by the fact that AIDS is now the leading killer of young men between the ages of 25 and 45. It is also the third leading killer of women in the same age group.[5]

Let's be clear about one thing. This disease is not limited to gay men or IV drug users. AIDS has often spread into innocent families by one marriage partner engaging in promiscuous behavior—heterosexual or homosexual—with someone who has AIDS. This individual can then bring the disease into his/her home and infect one's wife or husband and their unborn children. AIDS is ravaging people around the world in epidemic proportions.

Unfortunately, the public response to persons with AIDS has been close to hysteria. People have all kinds of fears about AIDS and do not know how to react. People often ostracize not only the person with AIDS, but treat the person's whole family with disdain. The closest biblical parallel seems to be the experience of leprosy. Leprosy, or Hansen's disease, usually took various forms. The most common form first began as a white speck on a person's body. The spot would begin to grow and slowly spread over the person's body until eventually his or her whole body would be completely white. Some forms of leprosy caused the persons to lose parts of their fingers, hands, or other parts of their body. Lepers were isolated from others, because people were afraid of contracting the dread disease.

Jesus and the Leper

Look for a moment at the story in the Gospels where a leper sought out Jesus (Matt 8:14; Mark 1:40-45; Luke 5:12-16). Matthew places this story right after Jesus finished the Sermon on the Mount. Matthew wrote first about the ideas and teachings of Jesus then noted his works and deeds. A crowd followed Jesus down the mountain. Suddenly the crowd saw the leper as he approached Jesus. They stopped, stepped back, and cried, "Unclean, unclean." But Jesus continued to walk toward the leper. The law forbade lepers to approach others. But the leper came near Jesus and cried out, "If you choose, you can make me clean." Jesus then reached out and did an unthinkable and unlawful thing in his day by touching the leper. "I do choose," Jesus answered. "Be made clean!" Immediately the leper was clean from his leprosy. Jesus told him to go and see the high priest and get the proper certification so that he could be declared clean and make the sacrifices the law required. Then Jesus said a strange thing, considering that a crowd of people was around him. "Say nothing to anyone."

AIDS and Leprosy

Some lessons in this story about the leper can give us some directions on how to respond to persons who have AIDS today. AIDS receives a similar reaction today to what leprosy received in biblical times. Certain of the responses in this story have parallels to our approach to those with AIDS.

An Attitude of Contempt

Notice in the Gospel story the contempt the people had toward a person with leprosy. "Unclean!" they cried. A person with leprosy was isolated from his family and other people. People avoided any kind of contact with him or her for fear of contracting the disease. It was said of a certain rabbi that, if he walked down a street where the shadow of a leper had fallen, he would not even eat an egg that a chicken had laid on that street. Some rabbis would throw stones at lepers to keep them away.[6] A leper was not supposed to come within six feet of another person. People dreaded lepers and isolated them. Many could not bear to look at them. Some people thought leprosy was a mark of sin. Leprosy was seen by these persons as the judgment of God on a person for something that individual had done. Do you remember the occasion in John 9 when Jesus was asked if the blind man or his parents had sinned? "Neither," Jesus said. "He was born blind so that God's works might be revealed in him" (John 9:1-3).

Some people are saying today (mostly televangelists) that AIDS is the judgment of God upon gay people. I do not believe that at all. What an awful concept of God that would be. This vindictive attitude is not the concept of God we have seen in Jesus Christ as the Father God who loves all persons. God cares for humanity so much that God sent His Son into the world to redeem it. Some people have such disdain for homosexuals and drug users who get infected that they moralistically assume that AIDS is God's judgment against them.

They say in so many words, "Well, it's just tough; they have AIDS. That's punishment for their behavior." But I do not believe for a moment that this would be the attitude of Jesus toward these people today.

The other side of the story about persons with AIDS is that it is not just gays or drug abusers who are getting AIDS. Tragically, some of those with AIDS are innocent children who contracted the virus from an infected mother. The mother may have contracted AIDS from a tainted blood transfusion or an unfaithful partner. Does God pick out innocent people to punish? I cannot believe it! God is not that kind of God. Jesus rejected this notion about God; so should we.

The Fayetteville (NC) Observer-Times carried a front-page story about a family infected with the HIV virus. Neither the husband nor wife was homosexual, and neither used drugs, but one of them contracted the virus from a former sexual partner. They do not know which one infected the other. The mother later had a child who was born with AIDS. "Life's too short for blame," Kim Starling said. "And it wouldn't change anything."[7] Does God cause things like this to happen to people? Of course not! The natural laws of the universe function so that exposure to the virus causes a person to contract the disease. If I come in contact with a cold virus, I likely will catch a cold. That is a law of nature. It is not God's judgment. Cancer, heart attacks, strokes, and other diseases, as well as the AIDS virus, function within the predictable, natural laws of the universe and are not the wrath of God upon people. We receive both good and evil reactions as we learn to cooperate or rebel against the world in which we live.

In the revelation of Jesus Christ, we have seen that God is a God of love. To assume that AIDS is the wrath of God seems to me to be more of an emotional response than a sound theological and biblical insight. How quickly some are to blame any kind of disease or plague on the wrath of God rather than on the natural function of our environment. The Bible reminds us that it rains on the just and the unjust.

Like the ancient leper, often people with AIDS are shunned, avoided, rejected, and isolated. Out of fear, people withdraw from them. As the Nazi Third Reich tattooed Jews during World War II and isolated them in concentration camps, many with AIDS have been treated as outcasts. A young man said that when he told his family he had AIDS, "They immediately kicked me out of the house. I felt like a leper." Like the ancient crowd's response to the leper in Jesus' day, contempt, fear, and hysteria are still very much with us.

The Cries of Pain

Notice that the leper cried out to Jesus, "If you choose, you can make me clean." The victims of AIDS are crying out all around us today. They face awful suffering and certain death. There is no known cure for AIDS. Death from this disease is usually painful and debilitating. When told they have AIDS, many of the victims cry out, "Why me? What have I done?" They sometimes ask, "Is God punishing me? Have I committed the unpardonable sin?" Those with AIDS go through the typical stages of people facing death—denial, anger, depression, bargaining, and acceptance.

But they also cry out wanting to know if there is anyone who cares. They feel ostracized, alone, and rejected. They sometimes struggle with whether to commit suicide. They sometimes are rejected from their own homes by their families. AIDS victims have anger toward themselves, their family, the person who gave them AIDS, friends, the church, society at large, government and even God. They suffer from psychological factors such as guilt, shame, fear, alienation, and low self-esteem. Most suffer from the stigma society puts on them, and they become victims of discrimination.

AIDS victims know many losses in their lives. They often lose their jobs. They suffer from a loss of direction in life, support, romance, love, trust, freedom, identity, meaning, purpose, security, and hope, or from growing old. They often suffer a loss of hospitalization insurance and even hospital accommodations. There have been cases in which a husband or wife has lost his or her job when it became known that the family had been touched by the AIDS virus. Sometimes AIDS victims suffer not only a loss of job but a loss of their church, friends, neighborhood, apartment, home, marriage, possessions, and financial security.

One of the saddest reactions to AIDS is to see a family turn against their own children. The young man I mentioned at the beginning had the good fortune of having his mother and brother stand by him. His father was dead. But his mother, brother, and companion remained with him until the end. He was one of the fortunate ones; others are often not so lucky. Many clothe themselves in secrecy to avoid rejection by family, friends, an employer, clients, business

partners or customers, ministers, or others. The circle that knows the
truth is often very small.

The Importance of Compassion

Notice the compassion of Jesus in this story. Many could not even
bear the sight of the leper, but Mark tells us that Jesus was moved with
compassion. Jesus consistently had concern for the outcasts. He
reached out to those who were hurting, rejected, a part of the outcast,
or the underdog in society. An old hymn entitled, "The Great
Physician Now Is Near," says it well:

> The great Physician now is near,
> The sympathizing Jesus;
> He speaks the drooping heart to cheer,
> Oh! hear the voice of Jesus.
>
> Sweetest note in seraph song,
> Sweetest name on mortal tongue;
> Sweetest carol ever sung,
> Jesus, blessed Jesus.[8]

Jesus showed compassion to this leper. He reached out to him and
touched him. Jesus indicated in his first sermon at Nazareth that his
ministry was to be directed toward the hurting, needy, rejected people
of society. He drew upon the words of the prophet Isaiah to foretell
his mission. In his commissioning sermon he said that he had come to
bring deliverance to the captive; to open the eyes of the blind; and to
help the lame to walk, the deaf to hear, the leper to be cleansed, and
the poor to receive the Good News (see Isa 61:1-5; Luke 4:16-21;
Matt 11:2-6).

Jimmy Allen experienced the personal tragedy of his grandson's
contracting HIV from a contaminated blood transfusion that infected
his mother and then was passed on to her son. Rather than finding a
compassionate response from churches, his family was shunned and
abandoned. In his book, *Burden of a Secret,* Allen challenges Christians
to show love, compassion, and healing as our Lord did by reaching
out to the untouchables of the first century.[9]

In the parable of the good Samaritan (Luke 10:29-37), Jesus
turned the pointer back to the lawyer, who originally raised the
question, "Who is my neighbor?" What was the lawyer's response?

"The one who showed him mercy." Neither the priest nor the Levite really showed concern. They were religiously proper, but did not want to get involved. They might be contaminated or inconvenienced. The one who was really a neighbor was not merely one who had a religious role or talked about religion, but one who put his words into action. The real neighbor is always the one who shows mercy.

The Contact Impact

Jesus did a surprising thing. He made contact with the leper. He touched him. Touching a leper was forbidden in that day. Could Jesus have cured the leper simply with a word? He had healed people before with just a word. His word could have been enough. But Jesus said, "I do choose." And he reached out and touched the leper. Lepers were supposed to keep their distance in biblical days. They were isolated, shunned, despised, and estranged (Lev 13:45-46). No one touched them for fear of getting the dreaded disease. Jesus touched the untouchable.

Many today do not want to touch people living with AIDS, out of fear of contracting the disease. People with AIDS are the contemporary untouchables. But Jesus reached out and touched the leper. The man had probably forgotten what it was like to be touched. He no longer had the touch of family, the embrace of his wife or children. He did not have the touch of someone pouring oil on his head to anoint him or to pour oil on his tired feet. There were no embraces from family or friends, yet Jesus reached out and touched him.

Ashley Montagu says that touch is "the mother of all the senses."[10] It is likely the first response we sense as a baby. Studies indicate that touch may be the last sense that dying people have. Touch! Touch was the vehicle Jesus used to express his love. Love will continue to use the sense of touch to communicate its message to others. Genuine love cannot remain at arm's length. It must embrace.

Several years ago when George Bush was president of our country, his wife, Barbara, visited Grandma's House on Logan Circle in Washington, D.C. This was a home established to house and support babies and young children infected with the HIV virus. These are innocent victims of drug-addicted parents. While Mrs. Bush was at the home, she walked around and hugged every single child in that place. She touched them all. The administrator of Grandma's House knew that the photos from the reporters who walked around with

Mrs. Bush would help correct some of the ignorance and prejudice people have toward people with AIDS.

Before she left, a thirty-nine-year-old man, who was head of the Damien Ministries, a Catholic organization that works with AIDS victims, came up to Mrs. Bush and thanked her for hugging the children. But he told her further that she might send the wrong message if she hugged only the babies. Innocent babies with AIDS need hugs; so do adults who have AIDS. Mrs. Bush didn't hesitate for a moment. She reached out and embraced him while the cameras flashed.

It is ok to touch people with AIDS. They are not the untouchables. They are persons who yearn to be touched and loved.

Complying with the Laws

It is interesting to observe that although Jesus did not hesitate to challenge much of the ritualistic laws of his day, he did encourage the man, who was clean of his leprosy, to go and get the proper certification from the priest. He urged him to comply with the medical practice of his own day. He directed this man to complete the necessary tasks to be officially declared clean.

Today we ought to work with the medical profession and other groups that are seeking to find a cure for AIDS. I still believe there is hope for finding a cure or a vaccine for inoculation. God is working through medical science, government, education, and other resources to find a cure that has not yet been found for this dread disease. There is one. Science seems to be closing in on this elusive and complex virus. Today it ravages the earth; tomorrow it will be controlled by a vaccine.

The Role of the Church

Meanwhile, the question is how the church is to confront the problem of AIDS. What are you and I as Christians to do because of it? What role can the church take in combating this problem? Let me suggest a few things.

The Church's Problem

First, let us acknowledge that AIDS is the church's problem. It is not just the problem of science, medicine, law, or government. It is the problem of the church as well, because there are people in the churches who have AIDS. There are families in our churches who struggle with children or spouses who have AIDS. We are indeed, as Letty Russell reminds us, the church with AIDS.[11] AIDS is our problem, too.

As a Baptist minister in Florida, Bill Amos led his church to confront the problem of AIDS in its own community. There were several people in his church with AIDS. The church's response is a dramatic lesson for all churches on how to minister to persons with AIDS. His book traces the steps of how ministry was provided to those in the church family who had this dread disease.

Amos suggests preaching and teaching with compassion about AIDS issues, equipping church members to minister to AIDS victims and their families, forming support and prayer groups, establishing policies for the church nursery, and providing hospice care.[12]

But the church's response has not always been positive. I read about a young man who had become a Christian while he was in the Kaiser Permanente Medical Center, and he wanted to be baptized by immersion. He made an appeal to a church nearby to use its baptistery to be baptized. The church refused. The members said he might contaminate the water, and others would get AIDS from him. Medical doctors assured the church members that this was not possible, but they still refused. Fortunately, another church happily allowed him to be baptized in its facilities.

The church needs to realize the immensity of the problem of AIDS. In October 1992, in Washington, D.C., a giant quilt was spread out in Memorial Park. It had more than 20,000 different panels on it representing persons who had died with AIDS. The quilt was longer than three football fields. More persons will die with AIDS. The problem is growing worse each day. The research of Dr. David Ho, *Time* magazine's "Man of the Year" (1997), and others has given some hope that a solution to eliminate or control the AIDS virus might be found one day. But scientists and physicians have not yet achieved that goal. We all pray it will come soon.

AIDS has come to the church. The church cannot ignore it. It cannot close its door and turn its back on the problem. It is inside the walls of our churches today. We are called to be leaders. Let us respond and not ignore this grave problem. We need to ask ourselves what our Lord would do.

At the Toronto Consultation on AIDS in October, 1987, which was jointly sponsored by the World Council of Churches and the

National Council of Churches in the U.S.A. and Canada, one study group delivered this powerful challenge to the church:

> The questions surrounding AIDS are often ambiguous and the answers often inadequate. Nonetheless, each individual and each church must struggle with this uncertainty. To do nothing is to make a profound statement about the nature of illness and health in our society. Silence can be deadly. Persons with AIDS and those with HIV infection are among us and not separate from us. The crisis of AIDS is our crisis. It is not a "we/they" issue. The church must share in this experience, changing and being changed so as to enable society to provide a supporting presence for those who are grieving and suffering.[13]

The AIDS National Interfaith Network offers help for local churches. It provides resources in education and guidance for meeting the crisis with compassion, support, nonjudgmental care, and personal assistance. The AIDS Action Council, the Centers for Disease Control, and other organizations can also provide useful information and help for churches.

Education

The church needs to educate our people. When I was a minister in Louisville, Kentucky, I served on the Louisville and Jefferson County AIDS Task Force. This group worked for a number of years. It was composed mostly of doctors and community health officials. I was the only minister on it. My eyes were opened to the immensity of the AIDS problem and how the churches in the past have often ignored the problem and refused to deal with it. The church needs to be engaged in providing education to fight the ignorance and hysteria that surround AIDS.

The church should educate people about how one gets AIDS. AIDS is contracted during sexual intercourse with someone who has the disease. It can also be acquired by using the drug needle of a person who has AIDS. An infected needle, for example, may be passed from one person to another. A person who has AIDS may stick the needle in her ear for an earring or use the needle for tattooing and pass that infected needle on to another individual who will become infected. A body builder who uses steroids might have AIDS and pass that same needle on to another person who uses the same needle.

AIDS is a blood disease and is passed on through blood or semen. It has been transferred through blood transfusions or from a mother with AIDS to her unborn baby.

AIDS is not an airborne disease. It is not a water disease. You do not get AIDS from mosquito bites. You will not get AIDS by drinking water or eating food after someone with the disease. You will not get AIDS from hugging someone who has the virus or even from kissing them. AIDS is not contracted by casual contact or by shaking hands with a person with AIDS. You will not get AIDS from their coughs or sneezes or from using their toilet seat. We need to know how AIDS is transmitted and end the hysteria and ignorance.

The church also needs to provide sex education. Christians should know that the human body is the temple of God. Sex is both beautiful and wonderful within marriage, but it is dangerous and risky outside of marriage. Promiscuity, adultery, and infidelity can be fatal. AIDS is a real, not a minor, danger. Sex education challenges Christians to honor the body that God has given us. Sex is beautiful in a faithful relationship in which one has bound himself or herself in marriage with the one he or she loves.

Too many persons have bought into the Hollywood and TV mentality that sexual activity has no real restrictions. This philosophy says, "It is ok to engage in sex with any and everybody, any place, any time, you feel like it and the two are consenting adults." This is a sinful and dangerous attitude. The first sex education our young people get should not be about AIDS. Our business is to tell of the wonder and beauty of sex within marriage and the importance of faithfulness in marriage. Let us say loudly and clearly that promiscuity and infidelity are sinful and dangerous in the world of AIDS.

Support Groups

The church needs to form support groups and not reject persons with AIDS nor their families. I have been in churches that have had widow, divorce, and grief support groups, as well as AA support groups. In some communities we need to establish AIDS support groups for persons with AIDS or families of those who have AIDS, because they often feel isolated or rejected. AIDS victims feel rejection enough. The church needs to treat them as persons and not objects. We may not agree with someone's lifestyle, but we can accept them and listen to them. We can hate the sin but love the sinner.

I read about a woman who got AIDS through a blood transfusion. When her husband discovered it, he left her. He had already lost his job when his company found out that his wife had AIDS. She gave birth to a child who had AIDS. She fled to another city. No one befriended her. She suffered from isolation. She could not find anyone who would support her.

Contrast that story with First Baptist Church in Plantation, Florida, where Bill Amos served as pastor. The church established support groups and ministered to AIDS victims and their families. One Sunday morning one of the women who had AIDS came down to the front pew where she usually sat. A dedicated church member, who was known by everyone in the church, came in a few minutes before the service began and walked all the way down to the front and hugged this person with AIDS and welcomed her back to church. By her act, she said, "I love and support you."

Persons with AIDS need our support. They are hurting. They need to know that the church cares. Ongoing support is essential for their families as well. According to Therese A. Rando,

> Despite its similarity to bereavement following other terminal illnesses, mourning associated with an AIDS-related death, incorporates greater-than-usual rage, fear, shame, and unresolved grief. The emotional damage caused to families by AIDS far surpasses those experienced in other of life's tragedies.[14]

Confidentiality

The church needs to maintain as much confidentiality as possible for persons with AIDS. According to current laws, HIV test results should be regarded as confidential medical information. This legal protection should be continued. Persons at risk, such as doctors, nurses, funeral directors, and pathologists, should be made aware of the dangers but keep the facts confidential. If a person's confidentiality is violated, that individual might lose his/her job and be ostracized by the community. Reporting and notification procedures and treatment should be done with confidential protection.

A Caring Community

The church needs to be a caring community. The church should work through Hospice or some other agency in the community to assist persons with AIDS or the HIV infection. Too many persons with AIDS have no family or anywhere to go. They are rejected and are all alone. If they can't go home, they need somewhere. Elizabeth Kubler-Ross, who has written many wonderful books about death and dying, tried to establish a sanatorium near her home in the mountains of Virginia for children who had HIV virus. Residents of the community protested loudly and blocked her efforts. They felt sorry for the children but did not want that home near them.

In the parable of the good Samaritan, Jesus tells us that the good Samaritan not only took care of the wounded man, putting himself in danger, but he also brought him to a hotel and paid for the cost of the lodging, food, and care. Jesus does not want us to reject people who have nowhere to go. Let us say to these hurting persons that we care and we love you, and want to find lodging for your needs. Let us work with the government, community, and health officials to find housing to meet the demands.

Some of you may have heard the story about Father Damien, the Catholic priest who went to a leper colony to minister. At the beginning of his ministry, he addressed his congregation as "you lepers." But after years of ministering among them, he contracted leprosy and then he would say tenderly, "we lepers."

We need to see that the people with AIDS are a part of the body of Christ. These people are human beings in need, and many of them are Christians, and Christians do not reject Christians or fellow human beings in need. Let us reach out to see how we can help them, and support them, and minister to them as we would with someone who has cancer, heart trouble, or any other kind of disease. We want to be supportive and loving like our Lord.

Following Our Lord's Example

We want to follow our Lord's example. We need to ask, "What would Jesus do? What would Jesus' response be to people with AIDS and to their families?" Would Jesus say, "I am going to reject you and have nothing to do with you"? I don't think you can demonstrate that response from the New Testament. Just as Jesus reached out and touched the leper, Jesus spent his life reaching out to those who were the underprivileged, the ill, the hurting, the blind, the deaf, the lame, the widowed—anyone in need. Whoever they were and wherever they were, Jesus reached out to minister to them. "Those who are well have no need of a physician, but those who are sick; I have come to call not the righteous but sinners to repentance" (Luke 5:31).

The Talmud, a collection of Jewish writings, tells a story about Elijah. A rabbi asked Elijah one day, "Where can the Messiah be found?" "You will find him at the gate of the city," said Elijah. "How shall I recognize him?" asked the rabbi. "He sits among the lepers," answered Elijah. "Among the lepers!" exclaimed the rabbi. "Why, what is he doing there?" "Changing their bandages," responded Elijah. "He changes them one by one."

Jesus will be ministering among people whatever their needs are. God's love is an inclusive love. Nothing separates us from the love of God no matter what it is. Nothing separates us from the love of God when we are in Christ Jesus, our Lord.

This was the word I shared with John Smith when he was frightened that he might have committed the unpardonable sin. The fact that he was concerned about it revealed he had not committed that sin. I encouraged him to accept God's acceptance of him. I assured him of God's grace and forgiveness and that nothing separates us from God's love—absolutely nothing—when we are in Christ Jesus our Lord (Rom S:35-39).

I wonder, if Jesus were telling the story of the prodigal son, might he not change it ever so slightly today? Maybe Jesus would have him come back and say to his father, "Father, I have sinned and I am no longer worthy to be called your son. I have AIDS, but I did not know where else to go." I think the father still would have welcomed him back. He would still say, "This is my son, who was lost, but has been found." He would have brought him back into his family, ministered to him, accepted him, and loved him.

On the day of judgment, Jesus says people will ask, "When did I give a cup of cold water in your name? When did I visit those in prison? When did I do some other service to you?" Jesus declares, "Just as you did it to one of the least of these who are members of my family, you did it to me" (Matt 25:40). To reject any person who has a need, no matter what that need is, is surely not like our Lord. When we look into the faces of those with AIDS, does not our Lord look out to us? Inasmuch . . .

Notes

[1]Letty M. Russell, ed., *The Church with AIDS* (Louisville KY: Westminster /John Knox Press, 1990) 43-44.

[2]Jimmy Allen, *Burden of a Secret* (Nashville: Moorings Press, 1995) 209.

[3]"International Projections/Statistics," *World Health Organizations,* 525 23rd Street, Washington DC.

[4]Center for Disease Control, *HIV/AIDS Surveillance Report,* June 1996.

[5]Morbidity and Mortality Weekly Report (U.S. Department of Health and Human Services, 16 February 1996) 45/No. 6.

[6]William Barclay, *And He Had Compassion* (Valley Forge PA: Judson Press, 1976) 35.

[7]*Fayetteville Observer-Times,* 6 March 1994, 1.

[8]William Hunter and J. H. Stockton, "The Great Physician Now Is Near," *Hymns for the Living Church* (Coral Stream IL: Hope, 1974) 71.

[9]Jimmy Allen, *Burden of a Secret* (Nashville: Moorings Press, 1995) 223.

[10]Ashley Montagu, *Touching* (New York: Harper & Row, 1972) 1.

[11]Russell, 152-53.

[12]William E. Amos, Jr. *When AIDS Comes to the Church* (Philadelphia: Westminster Press, 1988).

[13]Quoted in Russell, 43.

[14]Therese A. Rando, *Treatment of Complicated Mourning* (Champaign IL: Research Press, 1993) 634.

Suicide

Who is responsible? Can all the responsibility be placed at the feet of the genetic factors? Is the family "at fault"? What about situational factors?

The responsibility for suicide must finally be placed at the feet of the suicidal person. To do otherwise would be to deny the freedom of the individual. But does the individual act alone, and is he all-powerful to resist all the forces leading to suicide? No. Suicide and suicide attempts must be seen in the context of many contributing factors. A simple cause-and-effect explanation must be avoided. Every suicide and every suicide attempt speaks to us of the mystery and the complexity of life.

Because we are human beings who care, we bear the burden of responsibility. But there are limits to our responsibility.

Bill Blackburn
What You Should Know about Suicide[1]

There are many feelings associated with a suicide, and survivors need to be aware of them and work through them rather than become a victim of the suicide. The goal is to return to a wholeness of life as one builds for the future.

Perry H. Biddle, Jr.
Reflections on Suicide[2]

Many survivors of suicide carry a special burden throughout the process of grieving. Higher levels of guilt, shame, and anger are just three of the emotions that such survivors may experience. In addition, those grieving loss by suicide often are left with questions such as why their loved ones killed themselves and what, if anything, might have been done to prevent the suicide. Such questions, generally unanswerable, may prolong the process of grieving and condemn suicide survivors to live in the shadow of that suicidal death far longer than is healthy.

Kenneth J. Doka
Living with Grief after Sudden Loss[3]

The telephone rang; I picked it up. It was a church member who exclaimed, "Come quickly, Mrs. Blank has just killed herself." As I drove to her home and reflected on her death, I was not surprised. I had talked with her for some months, and she had been seeing a psychiatrist. I had warned her children to remove all guns and any other possible weapons from the home. But they had not taken her threats of suicide seriously.

When I was teaching at the Southern Baptist Theological Seminary in Louisville, Kentucky, I found a note at the bottom of one of the papers I had assigned to the students. The student wrote, "I have recently been contemplating suicide, but I have decided not to do it because it would not give me another chance."

Several years ago the theological world was stunned to read that Dr. Henry P. Van Dusen and his wife had committed suicide. He had been president of Union Theological Seminary in New York City and a leading teacher of ethics in our country. He left a note indicating that they were both increasingly weak and ill and did not want to live in a nursing home. Their suicide pact was the only exit they felt they had left to them.

When my son was in high school, he was a pallbearer at the funeral of a friend who had committed suicide. Following several years of heroin addiction, his uneasiness with fame, and personal problems, Kurt Cobain, at age twenty-eight, took his life and left a note saying,

> I haven't felt the excitement for so many years. I felt guilty for so many years. The fact is I can't fool you, any one of you. The worst crime is faking it.[4]

In our own community, the suicide of a fourteen-year-old Littlefield Middle School student was a shock to the city of Lumberton, North Carolina. Over the years, I have been called upon to minister to a number of church members when one of their family members has committed suicide. One of the most difficult of these experiences was helping the family of a young mother who killed her seven-year-old son and then turned the gun on herself.

A Major Problem

Suicides are a major problem in our country. Forty thousand people a year commit suicide in the United States. The real figures may be even higher, because experts are not sure how accurate the records are. In some areas of the country the figures are not gathered very reliably. In California, for example, until recently, unless a person left a suicide note, that person was not listed as a suicide—and of course, not all people who commit suicide leave a note. Annually, more than a million people in the United States attempt suicide. Among people over age sixty-five, especially widowers, suicide is a leading cause of death. Among college and high school students, it is the second leading cause of death. Suicide is one of the top ten causes of death in our country. In spite of this, many want to avoid talking or dealing with suicide. The church, of all places, should attempt to address this issue and offer guidance and help to our people.

The Scriptural Context

The word "suicide" does not appear in the Scriptures. Only six suicides are recorded in the whole Bible. In the Old Testament, King Saul was the most prominent individual who took his life. He died by falling on his sword rather than allowing himself to be taken captive by his enemies. After seeing the king kill himself, his armor bearer committed suicide also (1 Sam 31:1-6). Samson was captured, blinded, and mocked by the Philistines. Later, after his strength returned, he pushed down the support pillars of the temple, an act that caused the building to fall down killing him and all his enemies (Jgs 16:28-31). There are three other Old Testament characters whose suicides are recorded: Abimelech (Jgs 9:54), Ahithophel (2 Sam 17:23), and Zimri (1 Kgs 16:18). In the New Testament, the only suicide mentioned is that of Judas Iscariot. After he betrayed Jesus, he went out and hanged himself (Matt 27:3-16).

A Violent Age

I'm not sure that we should be so surprised at the prevalence of suicide in our country. After all, we are a violent nation. Violence is depicted as almost normal all the time on television and in the movies. Children and youth in some of our schools now carry guns and knives for protection. Violence looms all around us in the constant threat of war. Many of us drive violently on the highways, and accidents on the highways are one of the leading causes of death in our country. Some specialists in suicide are convinced that many of those who die in highway accidents show, by the way they drive all the time, strong suicidal tendencies. Likewise, some of us who work ourselves to death may be revealing some latent suicide motive.

Reasons People Commit Suicide

Why do people commit suicide? For some of us, it seems almost impossible to comprehend how anyone would want to take his or her life. And yet most people, at some time or another in their lives, have at least a fleeting thought of suicide. What are some of the reasons for suicide? There are many motives, but I will list just a few.

A Desire for Attention

Some persons attempt suicide as a cry for attention. Not everyone who attempts suicide really means to end his or her life. Sometimes it is an endeavor to get attention. "Hey, you wouldn't pay any attention to me when I was alive, so now maybe, by this act, I can get your attention." "Look at me." "I am here." "Take me seriously," they cry. Suicide may be a desperate gesture for help. "Pay attention to me," they scream. Any attempt at suicide is a loud cry for help.

In talking with one mother who asked if a suicidal attempt in her son was "just to get attention," Wayne Oates told her that her son had her attention with a bad report card. Now he wanted to know if she loved him! He had her attention. Underneath her comment about attention was the real question: "Should I take this gesture seriously?" And we must!

A Feeling of Being Unloved

Others commit suicide because they feel that they are unloved and unwanted. A college student looked up at me and said, "There would be absolutely no one—no one who would know if I were not alive. There is no one any place, anywhere that cares for me at all." There are many who feel unloved and unwanted, and they live out their lives groping and searching for someone to express some kind of affection for them. Many find their need for affection through pets. Animals become something to love and show affection to them.

Life Seems Futile

Others commit suicide because they have come to feel that life is absolutely futile. They see no point in living, and they are hopelessly frustrated. They feel like they have come up against a blank wall, and, no matter what they do, it is hopeless. "What is the point of it all?" they ask. The most dangerous emotion of all is, according to Paul Quinnett, "the state of hopelessness." "To be without hope is to be despairing of any future, of any relief, any cure, and of any promise that things will ever change for the better."[5]

Marsha Norman, in her play entitled *Night Mother*, depicts a young woman who had come to a hopeless perspective of her own existence. She felt that her life would only continue to be an empty, sad, pointless routine. Life was only futile for her. If her life continued, it would only be more of the same as before, and that was more than she could bear. She very rationally plotted her own suicide. She informed her mother of her intent and instructed her mother what to do after she had closed her bedroom door and shot herself. Life was too futile; so, she chose not to go on. Although the mother tried vainly to change her daughter's mind, she was unsuccessful.

In one of Charles Schultz's "Peanuts" cartoons, Sally is happily jumping rope. She continues to jump in two of the frames, but, then, suddenly she stops and starts crying. "What's the matter, Sally?" Charlie Brown asks. "What happened? Why are you crying?" "I don't know," she says. "I was jumping rope. . . . Everything was all right. When . . . I don't know . . . Suddenly it seemed all so futile!" Even through his cartoon strip, the pop theologian Schultz declares that some people experience only a sense of futility in life.

To Escape Pain or Disease

Some persons commit suicide because of their attempt to escape some dread disease. They do not want to have a lingering death filled with suffering and pain from their illness. Suicide is an avenue of escape for them out of what appears a hopeless battle with disease. When I was a graduate student in seminary, the whole campus was shocked when we received word that an Old Testament professor had killed himself. We gathered together as a community in chapel for his funeral, and I can still remember to this day the words Dr. Weatherspoon shared in his sermon about this professor who had ended his life rather than face the cancer from which he was slowly dying. For some, suicide is a way to avoid disease or illness.

To Avoid Disgrace

There are others who take their lives in order to avoid disgrace. They end their lives because they cannot face the disgrace of a failure in business, a marital affair that might be exposed, or something else. Rather than be disgraced, they remove themselves from life.

A Feeling of Guilt

A nagging sense of guilt is the reason some others take their lives. Judas struggled within himself over his own sense of guilt in having betrayed Christ. He felt such remorse that he threw down his thirty pieces of silver, and then went out and hanged himself. Some people cannot get over some sinful act they may have done or something they have *not* done. Their guilt becomes so strong because they have not found forgiveness, and they take their lives.

To Punish Themselves

Sometimes people commit suicide because they want to punish themselves. They have committed a wrong in the past, and since they have not been punished for it, they decide to punish themselves. Suicide is often an act of hostility which is turned inward. Karl Menninger views suicide as the wish to kill, the wish to be killed, and the wish to die.[6]

Several years ago a young teenager and his girlfriend went for a drive near Menlo Park, California, and accidentally ran into the rear of a tractor trailer truck. The young sixteen-year-old girlfriend was killed instantly. The young man later confessed that he had a little beer and marijuana. It only took a few weeks for his external scars to heal, but internally he was deeply damaged. When he went to the court hearing, his attorneys told him to plead not guilty. He became very angry when he could not plead guilty. "I took a human life, and you don't know what that means," Bobby told his family. Six weeks after his girlfriend was killed, he took his own life. He left a note to his girlfriend's parents. "I couldn't live without your daughter," he wrote. "When my carelessness took her away from me, I just couldn't stand to live without her." He asked his parents to bury him beside Joanne, "or I won't be happy," he wrote. Since he did not think the courts would give him the punishment he felt he deserved, he decided to inflict his own punishment.

To Punish Someone Else

Some persons commit suicide to punish the survivors. The hostility that had been directed inwardly is now directed toward others. "You wouldn't pay any attention to me in this life," one young man said, "so I will get even with you." "You don't show your love to me," another said, "so I will get back at you." The message they are sending to their parents is "I'd rather be dead than live with you. You will be sorry when I'm gone for the way you treated me." A father went out to get his morning newspaper and found the body of his daughter with a note that read: "I have come home, Daddy." Sometimes people take their lives to try to punish others whom they feel have hurt them.

Do Not Want to Be a Burden

At times persons commit suicide because they do not want to be a burden to others. They feel that their illness may be so long and costly that, like Dr. and Mrs. Van Dusen, they choose to take what they believe is a quicker and more inexpensive way. They fear that their illness will involve years of giving, and this will be a severe drain on their family.

Life Seems Meaningless

Others commit suicide because they have no sense of meaning in life. All purpose for them is gone. As the young man asked, "If you can give me any reason why I should go on living, I will." For many people who commit suicide, life seems to have no direction, purpose, or meaning. They have come to a dead-end street. They feel there is no one they can trust. Absurdity and despair fill their days. They have lost their perspective, their judgment is impaired, and they have lost their sense of humor. They suffer from a distorted view of life and cannot see their way clearly.

In some ways, suicide is a very selfish act. Persons become so entrapped with their own needs that they cannot see anything beyond them. Everything is judged by its effect on them. King Saul was enamored with himself, and he had consistently judged everything by what it did to satisfy his own ego. As he faced death, his primary concern was not to live but that his enemies not make sport of him. Many become so enamored with their own problems in life that they cannot see beyond them.

Myths

There are many myths or false assumptions that circulate about suicide. Remember, suicide is not the unpardonable sin. Like any sin, God can forgive it. Like any other mistake we make in life, we can trust God's love and grace. It is not true that all people who commit suicide always forewarn others first. Many times they do, but not always. It is a myth that all who take their lives leave a note. The act of suicide is not necessarily restricted to the poor or the rich, but it crosses all spectrums in society. Another myth is that if a person talks about suicide, he or she will not do it. Rather, talking about suicide is a sign that they might carry through. Take seriously all talk about suicide. There are a lot of myths about suicide. Books such as *What You Should Know about Suicide* by Bill Blackburn, *After Suicide* by John Hewett, and *Suicide: The Forever Decision* by Paul G. Quinnett may help you understand how to deal with many of these myths. These books offer helpful guidance in other areas related to suicide, too.

Signs

Let me suggest a few signs we ought to watch for when we think someone we know or love may be struggling with the possibility of suicide. Remember, not any one or two of these signs indicate that these persons are suicidal, but a combination of them might indicate that this individual needs help. A loss of relationship can be very significant. A person may lose his or her job. A move to a new community can be very difficult, especially for children. A person may lose a spouse by death or divorce. Loss of relationships can be traumatic. Some people consider suicide when their ego-needs have been badly shattered. Watch for signs when a person has failed in business, in school, or in romance. Any of these events can trigger deep emotional reaction.

Watch for prolonged acute depression that may indicate a need for professional help. Sudden changes in behavior patterns, moods, communication patterns, sleeping or eating patterns are signs of such depression. Watch for verbal clues such as: "I hate life, and I'm calling it quits." "I'm a failure." "My family would be better off without me." Being isolated and withdrawn and/or failure to communicate may be other signals to observe. A combination of these or others may indicate the need for professional help, and we ought to try to guide a troubled person to find that help.

How to Help

What can you and I as Christians do to help someone in our own family or a friend who might have some problems related to suicide? Let me make a few brief suggestions. One is very general, but I think it has prolonged implications for the impact it can have on the lives of people.

Be Sensitive

Learn to be sensitive to other people. I am convinced that one of the most devastating things with which we have to live is the insensitive and uncaring attitude that others direct toward us. Sometimes we experience insensitive behavior from professional people such as teachers or employers. Even peers treat us insensitively.

In devastating ways, children or teenagers constantly put down and ridicule each other. "Hey, skinny," they shout. "Moose." "Four-eyes." "Look at birdbrain." With words such as these, they belittle other persons. They do not begin to imagine how that devastates others. We all know what it's like when somebody hurts our feelings.

When we say something cruel or to hurt another person, think what that does to them. Some people never really get over what others say or do to them. Peer pressure can be devastating because of what it does to make another person feel rejected, isolated, unwanted, and unloved. Some parents constantly ridicule their children. They never give a word of praise to their children but always express ridicule, criticism, or blame. There is never a word of affirmation, appreciation, or love.

As Christian people, we need to say very clearly and simply that this demeaning attitude is not Christian. Christians should seek to affirm one another, to express love, and to be Christlike in all relationships. Teasing and unkind remarks can be crushing. We as Christians need to work hard to overcome that kind of negative behavior. If you are the victim of those verbal abuses, ask yourself, "Why is someone doing that to me?" I learned a long time ago that one of the reasons people act that way is because they themselves feel very insecure. They ridicule others and put another person down because in some way it seems to make them feel superior. This is a sign that they really feel inadequate. Remember, when you are the victim of someone else's ridicule, that individual may be a rather weak person. Try not to take the verbal abuse so seriously. To those who are tempted to ridicule another, remember that everyone is far more sensitive than you think. Instead of hurting them with your words, learn to express love, grace, and care to them. Being sensitive to them will be far more constructive than negative behavior.

Listen

Learn to listen to other people. Sometimes teenagers commit suicide because they can find no one who will listen to them. They cry out in every way imaginable to their parents and friends: "Listen to me; I've got a problem. Let me tell you about it." Husbands, wives, and friends reach for someone to take a few moments with them so they might communicate their frustrations. "Let me share with you the problems I am struggling with in my business or home," they say. "Let me tell you about this or that." When we learn to listen to each other, we extend a willing ear that communicates to them, "Hey, I care about you enough to take a few moments and listen." Listening telegraphs an important message to another person. It says we care for them and take them seriously enough to want to hear their pain, hurts, sorrow, or joy.

Seek Professional Help

When you are attempting to listen to a troubled person, if you pick up any serious signs of depression or other signals, direct the person to a professional for help. There are numerous resources in every community. You might call the Suicide Prevention and Education Center or the Crisis and Information Center. Many churches have full-time staff counselors who can assist. Individuals may sometimes need the professional help of a physician, psychiatrist, or pastoral counselor.

If persons have a need for trained professional help, please refer them without hesitation. To seek professional help with an emotional or mental problem does not indicate a lack of faith. If someone has a physical problem and you advise that person to see a medical doctor, do not think for a moment that this means this person does not have enough faith. They go to a physician to receive help in meeting a physical problem. If they have some emotional or mental illness, you should refer them to a doctor, psychiatrist, or counselor who can assist them in finding a cure for this type of illness. Like any other doctor, these professionals want to help you feel better.

I heard of a young woman who went to a football game in Nashville, Tennessee, several years ago. She had struggled with depression for some time and had been taking medicine that had helped. Unfortunately, she forgot to take her medicine with her. While she was waiting at her motel for her friend to pick her up, she began to feel nervous and upset. She called the Suicide Prevention Center, and the volunteer who answered the phone arranged for her to go to the emergency room at Vanderbilt Hospital. The psychiatrist on duty was able to give her the necessary medicine for the weekend.

Some forms of depression can be helped. Seek out those who are trained to give assistance. Let's not stigmatize those who suffer from mental trauma. Everyone who thinks about committing suicide is not mentally ill. These are people who need help. Do not be afraid to direct them to those who can help them. And, if you need help, do not be afraid to seek assistance from those who are trained to provide it.

Touch

Touch your friends with your support and concern. When I say touch them, I mean literally embrace them, hug them, and undergird them in their time of need. This message is especially needed in the relationship between parents and their children, children and parents, or husbands and wives. The child longs for the hug of a parent; an older parent needs the embrace of a son or a daughter; a wife longs for the arm of her husband to sustain her. A loving touch may help them through a tough moment.

A husband wrote about an experience when he had come to the lowest moment of his life. One night his wife awoke to see him weeping in a broken condition she had never witnessed before. His work had taken him away from home, and he had always been separated from her when he was torn apart by his inner fears. For the first time she saw him, with his guard down in his crisis moment. While he was sobbing uncontrollably, she reached over, and, without saying a word, took his head in her arms and drew him down against her breast. He sobbed as he had never sobbed before as though his soul was pouring out through his tears. "That was the moment," he said, "I have to thank for the fact that I am still alive, that moment when I was rocked and loved and comforted like the baby I had become."[7] This touch in a moment of deep need was therapeutic. Touch someone when they need you.

One of the significant traditions in the Old Testament was the passing on of the blessing by the father to his son. The son would kneel before his father, and the father would reach out and place his hands upon the son's head and pass on a blessing to him. How many children hunger for, long for, and grope for some parent to pass on their blessing to them? They want to hear their parents say, "You're ok; I love you." "There is nothing you can do to alienate yourself from my love." "I care for you."

Every child has a deep longing and hunger for a sense of touch both literally and verbally from their parents and others. Express your love to your children, wife, husband, parents, or friends. Tell them that you love and care for them. Express your love with an embrace. No matter what they may have done, don't reject them when they are in their lowest moment. Help them to come back from their seemingly bottomless pit. Express your love. Stick with them. Let them sense that you care for them and will be with them to the end.

John Bonnell was counseling with a businessman who had gone into a deep state of depression and felt his life was futile. The only thing that gave much satisfaction in his life was some exotic flowers that he cared for tenderly. He would work an hour each day nursing his exotic plants. Dr. Bonnell had gone out of the country for three months. On his return, he received a telephone call from the man's wife who indicated that her husband had slipped into an awful low state while he was away. She observed that she was afraid he would commit suicide. So Dr. Bonnell called him and asked if he could come by. The businessman agreed reluctantly. He found the man deeply depressed. He wondered what he could say to him. He simply sat there for a long time until he noticed that the man exotic flowers appeared to have gone uncared for. They were bone dry, and some of the leaves had withered.

Without saying a word, he began to pick off the dead leaves and blossoms. And then he began to work up the dry soil and poured water on the flowers. He worked for about fifteen minutes, and the man had not made a single move. Then suddenly, Dr. Bonnell noticed that a shadow crossed his path and his friend appeared with a vase of water and joined him in his task. In that moment, Dr. Bonnell felt that there was hope for his friend. They continued until they had watered all the flowers. Taking Bonnell's hand, his friend said:

> Thank you. From my heart I say thank you. I caught all the over-tones of what you have done. As I watched you picking off those dead blossoms and leaves, I knew that you were picking the dead leaves off my life. And like those plants, I feel that I have begun to live again.[8]

Express Your Love

Stick with your friend or relative. Assure your relative or friend of your support. Express your love. Your love can be expressed in simple ways. Sometimes you might help them do something around their house. You can express your concern by bringing them something tangible such as a book. Or if you cook, you might take them some kind of food. You might help them make plans for a trip or some project. Help older people in particular to find something creative to do. There is nothing worse than staying home and feeling as if there is nothing to do. For someone to think, "I am useless and nobody cares," is a bad state of affairs. Help them find something creative to do with their time and gifts. Through organizations such as senior citizen clubs, they might take trips and fellowship together. The church always needs someone to help make telephone calls or visits. Assure persons of the importance of prayer. Everyone can pray for others. Get older persons involved in some kind of activity or group so they may venture beyond the one room or two rooms where they spend most of their time.

God's Presence

But as Christians, above all, remember that we have resources from God upon which we can always draw. No person, no matter how low he or she may be in life, is totally without a resource for hope, because there is a God who loves us and cares for us. If you feel today that there is no one anywhere who loves you, know that God loves you. Do not lay down this book without hearing that God loves you. This is the great message we have from God through Jesus Christ. Suicide is not the answer. God loves you. God can bring you through the darkest valley of life. God is there with you in these dark places to sustain you and direct you through them. Do not give way to despair. Do not give way to depression. Seek help, but most of all be assured that God is present with you in your moment of need.

One of the great preachers in this nation was Harry Emerson Fosdick who was pastor for many years at Riverside Church in New York City. When he was a young man in seminary, he was involved in inner city mission work. He had worked so hard in his studies and mission work that he had a breakdown. He had suffered days and nights of sleepless tension, and a suicide attempt was prevented by his father. He was hospitalized for four months but was still not well. He took six more weeks away from his work and studies before he later returned to Union Seminary. During his senior year at Union, he became an associate minister at Madison Avenue Baptist Church in New York City. He later wrote in his autobiography about the years of struggle with mental depression and his inability to cope with the situation. The harder he struggled, the worse things seemed to get. Unable to deal with the situation, he learned a lesson that no seminary could ever teach.

> I learned to pray, not because I had adequately argued out prayer's rationality, but because I desperately needed help from a power greater than my own. I learned that God, much more than a theological proposition, is an immediately available resource.[9]

In his lowest moment in life, Fosdick found the presence and power of God to sustain him.

Today if you have any thought about suicide, remember that God loves you and God can help you to find the strength to overcome your depression and gain a positive perspective on life. Look to your family and friends; let them support you. Seek professional assistance. If you know anyone who may be contemplating suicide, assure them of your love and support and God's love. Guide them to find professional help. Remind them that God is with them and that God loves them. God has promised us that God's presence will be with us in the darkest of nights and the deepest of valleys. Draw on the strength of God's presence. Trust your life to God.

Notes

[1]Bill Blackburn, *What You Should Know about Suicide* (Waco TX: Word, 1982) 146.

[2]Perry H. Biddle, Jr. *Reflections on Suicide* (Fort Lauderdale FL: Desert Ministries, Inc., 1992) 22.

[3]Kenneth J. Doka, ed., *Living with Grief after Sudden Loss* (Bristol PA: Taylor & Francis, 1996) 50-51.

[4]*The Robesonian*, Lumberton NC, 11 April 1994, 5A.

[5]Paul G. Quinnett, *Suicide: The Forever Decision* (New York: Continuum, 1987) 74

[6]Karl Menninger, *Man Against Himself* (New York: Harcourt, Brace, and World, 1966) 50-80.

[7]Percy Knauth, "A Season in Hell," *Look* (19 January 1972) 76.

[8]John Sutherland Bonnell, *No Escape from Life* (New York: Harper & Row, 1958) 120-21.

[9]Harry Emerson Fosdick, *The Living of These Days* (New York: Harper and Brothers, 1956) 75.

From Shadows to Light

Aging

Being a child means growth, learning, developing, maturing. Adulthood means childbearing, and -rearing, the time of work. What comes next? The answer for most people, until relatively recently, is that they die. But when you realize that there are as many people alive over 65 years of age in the world today as in all previous history put together, you get the idea that the opportunity to grow old—to live into a new third age of life—has only rarely existed before. Now it is common and becoming more so, as 15 percent of women and 4 percent of men now live into their nineties. The most rapidly growing segment of the American population is the centenarians.

Walter M. Bortz
Dare to Be 100[1]

Recent research offers proof that even people of advanced ages who keep involved in life and maintain good health need not suffer a decline in creativity and intellectual capacity. Warner Schaie of Penn State University has been studying 3,000 people for decades, some of them now in their eighties. "For some mental capacities," he has said, "there begin to (be) slight declines in the 60s and more meaningful declines in the 80s. But some mental capacities decline very little, or can improve in old age." What counts is one's attitude toward life. "The expectation of a decline is a self-prophecy. Those who do not accept the stereotype of a helpless old age, but instead feel they can do as well in old age as they have at other times of their lives, don't become ineffective before their time."

Another study of this issue was made by the National Institute of Aging. Scientists there did brain scans of men ranging from twenty to eighty-three. They found that the healthy aging brain is as active and efficient as the healthy young brain. The conclusion was that although some brain cells are lost through the years, there are still more than enough functioning at an advanced age. It is a myth about aging that the years bring on senility. Senility is a result of brain disease, not part of the aging process.

Frank Hutchison
Aging Comes of Age[2]

When Booth Tarkington, the writer, was 75 years old, he was asked whether old people felt old in spirit. "I don't know," he replied. "Why don't you ask someone who is old?" Who are the old? We are all aging every minute, every hour, every day, every year. We either advance in age, or we die. How many of us ever pause to give thanks that we are growing older? But if we did not grow older, we would still be an inarticulate, dependent infant in the crib. No one desires that. The title of Sharon R. Curtin's book, *Nobody Every Died of Old Age*, says it well. An 80-year-old man I knew used to respond to the question, "How are you today?" with a twinkle in his eye, as he said: "I never felt better at this age in my life." You may die from cancer, a heart attack, or an accident, but old age itself will not be the killer. As long as you are alive, you are in the process of growing, maturing, and advancing in age.

One of the great myths of our time is that when a person reaches age 65 or 70, he or she is obsolete. According to the 1996 U.S. Bureau of Census, 31,000,000 people in America are over 65. In other words, 1 in 8 Americans is 65 or older. In fact, 1,000,000 people are over 90; of that number, 52,000 are more than 100 years old, and on their birthday each year, they receive a telegram from the president of the United States. The number of persons 65 or older was 10 times greater in 1990 than it was in 1900. The population of those 65 or older grew by 22% during the 1980s.[3] According to Lydia Bronte in a book entitled, *The Longevity Factor*, 85% of the 31,000,000 Americans over 65 today are active. Some 3,500,000 are employed, and millions are still productive.[4]

The number of persons in the United States who are past 100 years old is increasing all the time. Most of us hope to join that group some day. Some of us are closer to 100 than others. But think 52,000! In a study made of these persons, it was discovered that most of these people were still alert and active. A few of them could not see or hear as well as they used to, but most of them were still seeking to do creative things in life. Daniel Perry, director of the Alliance for Aging Research in Washington, D.C., observed, "Start rethinking your ideas about who's old." The centenarians are helping to stretch our sense of human potential. If people live to 100, how can you think of a person as being "used up" at age 65? We're approaching the day when 70 or 80 will be considered middle age.[5] We need to rethink the whole process.

More and more of us are getting older every day and living longer, and with the decline in the birth rate, the population is sloping in the opposite direction. The time of the "youth cult" is passing. We are entering into a new arena where the young no longer will be the predominant group in our society.

An examination of the attitude of today's society reveals what Paul Tournier has called a "great contempt" for the elderly. In his book, *Learn to Grow Old*, Dr. Tournier indicated that this contempt may not always be open or brutal, but it may range from haughty disdain to secret scorn.[6] This disparagement against the old may take various forms. Television and magazine advertisements declare, "Hate that gray? Wash it away!" "Feel young again." "Feel like a bride again." Society says, "Don't show your age." Use the proper soap or the correct makeup or wrinkle cream or get a face lift. Do anything to avoid revealing that you are aging. The youth emphasis is so strong that it appears to be a curse for one to show signs of getting older. Most persons seem to be open to acknowledging that they are aging until they reach 30 or 40, and then, they begin to deny or disguise the fact that they are aging.

In his book, *How to Stay Younger While Growing Older*, Reuel Howe relates an experience he had with a man in his mid-30s at a conference. "What are you doing here?" the younger man asked him. "Why, what do you mean?" Dr. Howe responded with surprise. "Why shouldn't I be here?" "Because you are so much older than the rest of us," he replied. "What do you expect to get out of this workshop?" "I'm here because I want to grow," Dr. Howe said, "to keep my juices flowing." "But how can you do that when you're so old?" the young man asked. As the conference continued, Dr. Howe said he was able to detect reasons why this man's attitude was so hostile toward his presence. Like so many in our society today, he had contempt for those who are older because of his own fear of aging and his own unconscious fear of dying. According to Howe, the "ghetto of age" has become a serious problem for contemporary America.[7]

Today's Attitude

The Chinese have a proverb that says, "The old are the precious gem in the center of the household." But this is not so in America. Society seems to say to the aging, "Move over and make room for those who are younger. Hurry up and get out of our way so we can take over and do things our way." In a recent study of employment, 97% of newspaper "Help Wanted" ads set 40 as the age limit. Similarly, 1/3 of employment agencies will not attempt to place workers over age 45. Forced retirement at 65 or 70 plunges many into idleness and others into destitution. Even if a person is still in full control of his or her reasoning and manual skills, society usually pushes him or her aside for a younger man or woman, as if youth alone will fill the vacuum of knowledge and experience.

The notion that the elderly have an automatic age at which they stop producing is nonsense and is challenged by recent studies. Oriental societies honor their elderly and seek out their wisdom. A recent White House conference on aging listed the following losses the elderly experienced:

•the loss of prestige
•the loss of authority
•the loss of income
•the loss of the home
•the loss of family and friends through death
•the instrumental role in society because of compulsory retirement
•the loss of time to do what one has failed to do or to undo what has been done in the past

The Elderly Are Alive, Too!

Attitude is a key factor in whether or not a person is old. A younger woman said to an older friend one day, "I wish I could grow old gracefully like you." "My dear," the older woman replied, "You don't grow old. When you cease to grow, you are old." A lot of us ceased growing when we were very young. At 18 some had their outlook on life set and have never changed it since. Even if they live to be 100, they will not be growing because they stopped responding to life when they were young.

To live to an advanced age is no guarantee of experiencing a meaningful existence. Methuselah, who is credited in the Old Testament with being the oldest living person, died at the age of 969. The only observation about his whole life is that he was the son of Enoch, had sons and daughters, and died. Longevity alone does not determine meaning. Some people fill fewer years with a great wealth of happiness and service. However, some people in their 80s are still alive and vibrant to life and live out their years with purpose, usefulness, and joy.

The book of Joshua contains a delightful story about a man named Caleb. At age 85, Caleb, who was one of the men sent by Moses to spy out the land of Canaan 40 years earlier, asked for his portion of the land that had been promised them. He declared:

> I am still as strong today as I was on the day that Moses sent me; my strength now is as my strength was then, for war, and for going and coming. So now give me this hill country of which the Lord spoke on that day. (Josh 14:11-12)

I like Caleb. Listen to him: "I am not old; give me another mountain to conquer. I am as strong as ever." Who knows whether he meant physical or mental strength? But what does it matter? His attitude was unconquerable.

My wife had an elderly aunt who until a few years ago kept old people in her home. She finally "retired" at 85, sold her home, got an apartment, and purchased herself a new automobile—her first one with power steering. She was still looking for another mountain to conquer.

A white-haired former school principal once said to a group of young people, "Have no fear of growing old. Old age is a rich and happy time of life. Life has still so much to offer. We can have peace within and joyfully look forward to the future."

Myths

A part of our fear of aging is a result of the misconceptions or myths that society portrays about the elderly. Who would want to be senile, unable to remember, lacking in mental skills, and without comprehensive judgments? In recent studies many of the stereotyped attitudes toward the elderly have been challenged.[8] Studies reveal that senility and intellectual decline are not automatically acquired when one turns 65 or 95. Few elderly people ever develop senility—only 1 in 6. Some do show senility that is caused by cerebral arteriosclerosis (hardening of the blood vessels) or atrophy (dying of the brain cells). For some, it is a result primarily of attitude. Society has conditioned many elderly people to assume they are supposed to become senile, and so some do. The notion of senility may well be one of the most damaging inventions of modern Western society to control the elderly.

Recent testing has indicated that a person has the same ability to learn at 80 as at 12. Dr. William Cole, professor of sociology at the University of Tennessee, declared at a conference on health and aging:

> While younger men and women may excel in motor activities, older men and women excel in tests on information, comprehension, and verbal skills. They also have the ability to profit from experience and have more natural judgment and wisdom.

Research has also indicated that persons over 65 are good employment risks, have greater work interest, experience, skill, and job attendance.

Another myth has it that when we grow older, our memories get worse. How often have we said, "Now that I am older, I just can't seem to remember"? Stop and think for a moment and ask yourself whether you ever had a good memory—even when you were young. Age, then, is not the reason we can't remember. For many of us, our memory has always been poor; it is not a condition we suddenly acquired when we became older.

Your Age Inside

In every single one of us there lives an old person and a young person. At times we let one or the other of these personalities out of our inner self more than the other. Our attitude can determine which one. Our lives are filled with varied experiences that have helped determine the person we now are. We are more than we think we are, yet less. We are constantly becoming; we are always growing, never still, never fully complete, never totally there, always en route. "I am large," said Walt Whitman, "I can contain multitudes." What shall we be, old or young? Our attitude determines which one we let out to play.

When I was in college, I remember a fellow freshman who seemed old at 19. He dressed, talked, and looked like a man in his later years. Why did he do this? Who knows? I know some people in their 80s who are delightfully young. Their attitude, their outlook, their interest, their activities make them younger than some of their con- temporaries in their 40s or 50s. When I look at the vigor and love of life that many of these elderly people demonstrate, I stand in amazement at some who have just turned 40 and feel they now have one foot in the grave. No one is ready for the pasture in their 40s, 50s, or older. Life may just be beginning for them.

I wouldn't trade places with the young people today for anything. I don't want to be a teenager again. I have learned so much since then. I know I have matured and have experienced life so much more deeply than I had at 16. No one should want to regress. Some of my friends in their 80s know so much more about life than I do. Their years have enriched them and made them more sensitive and knowledgeable. Those of us who are younger can learn much from them. Henri Nouwen observed,

> Aging is one of the most essential human processes, one that can be denied only with great harm. Every man or woman who has discovered or rediscovered his or her own aging has a unique opportunity to enrich the quality of his or her own life and that of every fellow human being.[9]

An elderly lady who was noted for her learning, grace, and hospitality once entertained a young student in her home. As the young man was leaving, he had been so charmed by her, and he searched for the right words to express his pleasure at being in her home. "I think you're perfectly beautiful," he said. "Thank you," she replied. "By this time I should be. I'm 70 years old."

Learning to Look Ahead

Aging is something that concerns all of us. As long as we are still living, then we are still aging. We must learn to live with it. Aging does not have to make us obsolete. The title of Jean Abernathy's book, *Old Is Not a Four-Letter Word!*, expresses a valid philosophy toward the elderly. All of us are on a journey through life from birth to death. To see life with a forward perspective and not as a deadend makes all the difference in the way we travel the journey. "At 80," Archibald McLeish, the poet, declared, "you have to begin to look ahead." We learn from the past, but we cannot live in it, nor are we anchored to it. The apostle Paul expressed it this way:

> I do not consider that I have made it my own; but this one thing I do: forgetting what lies behind and straining forward to what lies

ahead, I press on toward the goal for the prize of the heavenly call of
God in Christ Jesus. (Phil 3:13-14)

Whether we are 18, or 25, or 40, or 80, we cannot lock ourselves
into the rooms of the past, but we can experience real living as we
move toward the open door of the future. Life is still ahead of us, and
we are challenged to find the greatest meaning and purposes we can
within the time that lies ahead of us. Walter Bortz believes that our
aging should have as much creativity in it as possible. "Opportunities
for creativity vanish when risk taking is abandoned."[10]

Living with Aging

As you live with aging, consider some things that might enable you to
find a greater sense of meaning and purpose as you progress.

Accept Some Losses

Accept the fact that as we get older we become aware that there are
some things we may not do as well as we did when we were younger.
When we were young children, we looked forward to the time we
would be stronger and more alert mentally. After we pass our late 20s
or late 30s, our motor skills or strength might not be as strong as they
were in younger years. In the novel, *Growth of the Soil*, Isaac, a pioneer
who has spent his life using his physical power to clear and maintain
the land, finally became aware that he had grown older as he
attempted without success to remove a huge rock. He began to reflect,
"Am I getting old?"

As we get older, we do find that there are certain barriers that
change our lifestyle or manner of living. A man at 40 may not run as
fast as he did when he was young, nor can he play football as well as
he did when he was 20. At 80 our motor activities will not be the
same as they were when we were much younger. Sometimes we may
not see or hear as well as we did when we were 30. Glasses or a hearing
aid might help these conditions. Many older people, however, hate to
admit that they have a deficiency and so nothing can be done to
correct these problems.

A pastor friend of mine told me about a visit to his church by Dr.
Sydnor Stealey, the late president of Southeastern Baptist Theological
Seminary in Wake Forest, North Carolina. After Dr. Stealey had fin-
ished preaching, the pastor went to the door to greet the people as

they left while Dr. Stealey was speaking with members at the front of the church. An elderly gentleman, who was in his 90s and very hard of hearing, came out the door and remarked to the pastor, "I couldn't hear a word you said today, pastor." "Well, Mr. Jones," the pastor said, "I didn't preach today. Dr. Stealey from the seminary was our speaker. Why don't you go up and say a word to him?" "I think I will," he said. "I couldn't hear him at all." Addressing the seminary president, he said, "Dr. Stealey, I couldn't hear a word you said today. You should have spoken louder." Dr. Stealey, who was about 70 then himself, responded, "Old man, there is nothing wrong with my speaking voice. You are just deaf!" Then he put his arm around the man and hugged him and said, "You know, as I have gotten older, I can't hear so well either. I know what your problem is like." After that they talked freely for a while to each other with a mutual feeling of understanding and compassion.

Often we want to blame someone else when we can't hear or see as well or get some things done as quickly as when we were younger. Without question, aging does affect us in some areas. We have to learn to correct what we can and adjust to what we cannot.

Accept the Generation Gap

The generation gap is real. Pearl S. Buck stated in an article she wrote at age 80 that she believed in the generation gap. She strongly supported the practice of preserving the proper levels between parents and children, children and teachers, and young and old. What young people need are not buddies or pals from their parents or grandparents but models with leadership and concern. Pearl Buck observed,

> Only through the generation gap can each generation contribute its best; the young to use their impetuous zeal to learn and to progress, and the old to express their wisdom and optimistic belief in themselves. I have no wish to "be on the young side," advertisements not withstanding. I value my age. It took me a long, long time and much work to get where I am now. Shall I try, crabwise, to move backward? Not I! I believe in the value of old age and old people. I deplore the loss to our nation that we do not use this resource. I pity the foolishness of young people without wisdom and guidance, for the progress of the nation is impeded, slowed up, destroyed thereby. If each generation learns only by its own experience, we merely mark time and get nowhere. I am all for old people, myself

included, and have been so always. Anxious to learn, as a child and a youth in China, I sought out—not the young, for I knew what they had to say—but the old who had lived long before I was born.[11]

I remember a teenage lad telling me that he was attending a church that gave him and other young people an opportunity to stand up and preach to the congregation anytime they wanted to. I could not resist asking, "What do you know to preach?" At his age he has only begun to live and understand the experiences of life's meaning. Where did the idea come from that youth have the answers to the problems of humankind? Certainly young people need to be heard and have their say, but the experience of a lifetime from an older, informed adult can be invaluable.

Look to the Future

Accept a future orientation. It is normal for any of us to reminisce, but we can become so absorbed in our memories that we may miss the joy of living in the present. According to an old saying, "He who lives only in his memories is really old." To walk through the memory of our past can provide us with an opportunity for delightful reflections. But our primary stance is toward the future, not the past. We reflect on the past and are thankful for its blessings but face the future.

Lot's wife turned to a pillar of salt because she looked back. When we dwell only on the past and turn our attention to what is behind us instead of the possibilities that are still before us, then our potential for further growth has been curtailed. George Bernard Shaw stated:

> What makes us perceptive and gives us a sense of responsibility is not the number of years behind us but the number of years that are still ahead of us. Wisdom does not spring from our memories of the past but from our awareness of responsibility for the future.[12]

Enjoy Simple Pleasures

Accept the little joys of life. When we are younger, it takes much more to satisfy our quest for pleasure. Often the young want something to be gigantic, spectacular, or dramatic, or they are not satisfied in today's world. As we age, small things bring a deep sense of satisfaction and appreciation. If we do not take time to see the little "joys" around us, we may miss the beauty of a sunrise or sunset, flowers in bloom, buds bringing new life to our trees, our baby or grandbaby at play, time spent with our wife or husband, children or parents.

If illness has forced someone to be confined to bed, a visit from a friend brings a sense of remembrance. A letter from a loved one or friend, a cake baked by a neighbor, cut flowers from a friend's garden, a phone call from a relative or friend, a visit from the grandchildren, all these and others are occasions for little joys to so many who are elderly. Sometimes simply a good night's rest, a good meal, a warm room, a friendly smile, or an encouraging word can help those who are lonely and discouraged. We need to practice both giving and receiving these little joys of living.

Be Positive

Overcome pessimism and defeat. Reuel Howe declared:

> I try to avoid despair and pessimism because I recognize that they are killers. They kill hope, initiative, and a guiding purpose with which to keep life alive and moving toward a goal. To succumb to pessimism is a cop-out, to give way to deteriorating aging.[13]

Before anyone of us realizes it, we can get ourselves into a negative rut and be beaten down by a pessimistic attitude toward ourselves and others. The ancient writer is correct: "A cheerful heart is a good medicine, but a downcast spirit dries up the bones" (Prov 17:22).

In her helpful book, *A Crown of Glory: A Biblical View of Aging*, Rachel Z. Dulin provides a summary of the Bible's perspective on old age and spiritual experience. She notes:

> The biblical literature shows us that aging had physical and emotional components. As we have already observed, some writers conveyed the reality that aging was a process which brought decline to the body and caused great emotional distress and that it was a process which left one weak and vulnerable. Yet in the same literature we have heard the voices of those who thought that, in the complexity of human existence, aging should not be viewed only through the negating eyes of the beholder. Since to grow old was a part of the whole human experience, it should not be perceived only through its crippling consequences. To them it was "the crown of glory."[14]

No matter what the circumstances, all of us have a choice in determining what our attitude will be in the situation. We can choose to be gloomy and depressed or cheerful and optimistic. No one can avoid all difficult situations or problems, but we can decide whether we will meet them with assurance or defeat.

After a fire had destroyed their home and the only thing the family had left was the clothes on their backs, Dr. Howe relates how he and his father returned with supplies from a distant village to find that his mother had arranged a lunch for them on a log. In the middle of the log she had placed a rusty can filled with wildflowers. That was a powerful sign of optimism in the worst kind of conditions for them.[15]

I remember on numerous occasions how I would visit some of my church members who were elderly and bedridden with the thought that I might be able to cheer them some. But the reverse almost always happened. Many of those who lived with so much pain and difficulty still transferred radiance and hope to those who visited them. Maybe their inner strength enabled them to pass on to others something of their own power. I can still see Mrs. Jopes sitting on the front row of the church every Sunday. Although she was in her 90s and almost deaf, she never missed her hour of worship. She couldn't hear much, but she felt that it was her place to be in church on Sunday. Later when she was unable to attend, I would visit her and she would always give me a lift. She could not wait to recite the psalm or poem she had memorized. She always asked about the work of the church and the people. She continued to focus on the potential "we" still had as a church and the contribution "we" could "all" make in the community. She was still looking ahead.

Find Ways to Serve

Every church and community has a power source it usually overlooks. We might call it "senior power." Just a few years ago a thousand demonstrators marched outside the office of the governor of New York. But they were not college students. They were all senior citizens who were demanding increased benefits for the aged and disabled. Senior power provides the voltage for a host of ministries or the potential for them within every city.

Much of the ministry of our church and other churches is carried out by retirees. Many of these members have served in able places in our community before they retired, and their abilities have not lessened because they have reached the age of 65. They retired from one type of work to begin another. In my church our senior citizens serve in varied ways. They work on committees, visit and minister in nursing homes, carry sermon tapes to homebound members and the nursing homes, provide transportation, teach, do manual tasks, provide food for the Meals on Wheels program, and work in our mission causes and many other areas.

In smaller but equally important ways, words of encouragement and praise from the elderly can do wonders for children, youth, and even other adults. Several of the most exciting vibrant members of our church are in their 70s or 80s, and they are still filling meaningful positions of leadership and service.

Nurture Your Faith

Strengthen the foundation of your faith. Miss Curtin in her book, *Nobody Ever Died of Old Age*, tells about an old woman called Granny Suskie she met in a hill town in eastern Kentucky. Granny Suskie is over 100 and blind, but her step never falters. Granny Suskie said,

> The last years of a woman's life should be spent in trying to settle what's inside. Early on, a woman is so filled with things outside—her looks and her husband, and her children and her home—that she never has a chance to be just private. I've had more private time, now, than I need, but I value these years all the same.[16]

Everyone needs private time to strengthen the spiritual foundation of his or her life. No matter what our age is, no one has ever arrived spiritually. The more we learn of God and God's ways, the more we become aware of how much there is to know. Our spiritual life is one structure we are constantly remodeling. We build on the foundation we have and reach forward to what we can still become.

Find New Employment

If you desire, find a new job. There are some people who retire and then take another job. Another chapter of life may open up for you unexpectedly. One of the most delightful persons I know is Dr. Sarah Lemmon who taught history at Meredith College for many years. She retired at 65 and then for 10 years served in various administrative capacities at Meredith. She later moved to a retirement village in Southern Pines, North Carolina. She was always a very active

Episcopalian and began to work with the chaplain in the retirement home. At the encouragement of the chaplain, Dr. Lemmon, at 80 years old, was ordained a deacon in the Episcopal church. This is a professional ministry position. At 80 years old she continues to serve in this retirement village. I listened with great interest as she recently talked to a group of Meredith alumnae about her sense of call to ministry, and her training and preparation for ministry. At 80 years old she began a marvelous new chapter in her life. Who says that when one chapter ends, life is over? Find a new chapter.

Continue to Learn and Contribute

While an older person's motor activities may slow down, there is no reason why a person cannot continue to excel in other areas—and many have. The following is just a sampling.

- Golda Meir became the prime minister of Israel at 71.
- Konrad Adenauer was first elected chancellor of West Germany at 73 and served for 14 years.
- Forced to retire at 70 as football coach at the University of Chicago, Amos Alonzo Stagg coached for 14 more years at the University of the Pacific and was voted "coach of the year" at 81.
- Socrates was 80 when he took up the study of music.
- Grandma Moses began painting at 70 and was still painting beautiful folk art at 100.
- Goethe wrote Faust when he was 80.
- John Wesley preached until he was 88.
- At 83, Gladstone was elected prime minister of Great Britain for the fourth time.
- Ronald Reagan was elected president of the United States when he was in his 70s.
- Arthur Rubinstein was still making concert tours at 85.
- Sophocles wrote Oedipus Rex at 75.
- Mohandas Gandhi was in his 70s when he achieved his goal of independence for India.
- John XXIII was elected pope at 77 and revolutionized the Roman Catholic Church.
- Karl Barth was still writing theological works when he was in his 80s.
- Benjamin Franklin helped draft the Declaration of Independence at 69.

- Claude Pepper, in his 80s, served as a senator from Florida.
- Tennyson was 83 when he composed "Crossing the Bar."
- Leeuwenhoek was 88 when he discovered spermatozoa, blood corpuscles, infusion, and so on.
- Michelangelo was 89 when he painted his *Last Judgment.*
- At 84 Agatha Christie was still writing crime novels, including *Nemesis* in 1971 and *Elephants Can Forget* in 1972.
- Robert Stolz was still composing in his 90s.
- Pablo Picasso was still experimenting with new art forms until he died at 90.
- Frank Lloyd Wright designed buildings until he was 91.
- Bob Hope continues to entertain America in his 90s.
- Mother Teresa, in her 80s, still ministers to the poor and needy in India.
- Nelson Mandela was elected president of South Africa at 75.
- Harry Emerson Fosdick, minister for many years of the famous Riverside Church in New York City, authored more than 30 books and wrote a bestseller for young people when he was in his 80s.

In addition to the contributions of these listed, Thomas Edison, Norman Vincent Peale, George Burns, Lena Horne, Thomas Jefferson, J. C. Penney, Colonel Harlan Sanders, George Bernard Shaw, and hundreds more have been productive into advanced age. I remember also the energy that Dr. John Rosser used to have when he was pastor emeritus of a church where I was pastor in Virginia. In his 90s he was still writing, preaching, and teaching. He was active until he died at 96.

Frank Hutchison in his book, *Aging Comes of Age,* challenges persons, "NEVER RETIRE!" Find some work, volunteer or part time, to satisfy your survival instincts and your work ethic. He notes that a person may retire from a particular job or occupation but not from life, from work, or from involvement.[17] With so much still needed to be done in our nation and world today, those over 65 still have a vital contribution to make. Stretch yourself and find new places and opportunities to use your gifts and skills. Be proud of your age. There are many who need to learn from your years, wisdom, and experience.

In my church in Lumberton, North Carolina, some of our most active and faithful members in attendance, teaching, giving, and serving on committees are persons in their 70s and 80s. Two medical doctors in our community were recently recognized for their achievements. One of them, age 70, passed an examination that earned him recognition as a nationally certified correctional health professional. The other is a deacon and faithful member of my congregation who was recently selected in our city as the most popular physician. This doctor in his 70s still practices medicine and performs surgery.

Continue to Grow

Continue growing through the journey of life. Even if your health is not good—hopefully you will stay well, but even if not—keep growing. There are always some things you can do. Don't rest on your oars. Arnold Toynbee wrote,

> Nothing fails like worldly success. My study of twenty-one civilizations has convinced me that cultures are healthy only when they are creative. The civilization that solves its problems and rests on its oars has a sad future if it does not respond to the next challenge with a different answer.[18]

Toynbee's words are true for individuals, for institutions, and for life. Look for a new chapter. Look for a new opportunity. Don't simply rest on your oars. See what lies ahead of you. Keep growing.

Creative people seem to live longer than those who are not. All of us have the possibility of cultivating our own creativity and making our own contributions. You may not become rich or famous, but you can be open and responsive to life around you and within you. You can be alive and live every minute of your existence with meaning and purpose. Don't let anyone convince you that a person who is elderly cannot contribute to society or enrich it. The parade of persons I have just mentioned belies that. Robert Browning expressed his vision about later years this way:

> Grow old along with me
> The best is yet to be.
> The last of life,
> for which the first was made.
> Our times are in his hand.
> Who saith: "A whole I planned.
> Youth shows but half,
> trust God see all, nor be afraid."[19]

In closing his book, *How to Stay Younger While Growing Older*, Reuel Howe says that before he concludes a service of worship with the benediction, he likes to ask the people to turn and look at the door of the church building and ask themselves whether that door is an entrance or an exit. The answer can make a great difference. If the door is merely an "exit," then there is no future; but if it is an "entrance," then each one is taking the meaning of the worship experience with him or her and going with trust into the world outside.[20]

The door of your church or the door of your house can represent to you an exit or entrance. Let it symbolize your entrance way into a path that puts you on the way to living and growing daily in a more meaningful way. Join your voice with the ancient Caleb and proclaim, "I am as strong as I ever was. Give me another mountain to conquer."

Notes

[1]Walter M. Bortz, *Dare to Be 100* (New York: Simon & Schuster, 1996) 23.

[2]Frank Hutchison, *Aging Comes of Age* (Louisville KY: Westminster/John Knox Press, 1991) 61.

[3]Bureau of the Census and the National Institute on Aging.

[4]Lydia Bronte, *The Longevity Factor* (New York: Harper & Collins, 1993).

[5]Daniel Perry, quoted by Caryl Stern, "Who Is Old?" *Parade Magazine*, 21 January 1996, 5. See also Beth B. Hess & Elizabeth W. Markson, *Growing Old in America* (New Brunswick NJ: Transaction Publishers, 1991); and Letty Cottin Pogrebin, *Getting Over Being Older* (Boston: Little, Brown, & Co., 1996).

[6]Paul Tournier, *Learn to Grow Old* (New York: Harper & Row, 1972) 36ff.

[7]Reuel L. Howe, *How to Stay Younger While Growing Older* (Waco TX: Word Books, 1974) 11.

[8]See Paul B. Baltes and K. Warner Schaie, "The Myth of the Twilight Years," in *Psychology Today* 7, no. 10 (March 1974) 35-40; K. Warner Schaie and G. Labourie, *Life-Span Development Psychology* (New York: Academic Press, 1973) 91-92; Ken Dychtwald and Joe Flower, *Age Wave* (Los Angeles: Jeremy P. Taracher, 1989) 156ff.; and Zalman Schachter-Shalom and Ronald S. Miller, *From Age to Age: A Profound New Vision of Growing Older* (New York: Warner Books, 1995.

[9]Henri J. M. Nouwen and Walter J. Gaffney, *Aging* (New York: Image Books, 1976) 154.

[10]Bortz, 127.

[11]Pearl S. Buck, "What I Now Believe," *Family Weekly*, 13 February 1972, 7.

[12]George Bernard Shaw, source unknown.

[13]Howe, 43.

[14]Rachel Z. Dulin, *A Crown of Glory: A Biblical View of Aging* (New York: Paulist Press, 1988) 99. Frank Stagg, *The Bible Speaks on Aging* (Nashville: Broadman Press, 1981) explores the biblical view of aging, notes some of the stereotyping in the modern world, and affirms a positive attitude toward aging. A recent article entitled, "Researchers Shoot Down Aging Myths" by Leonard J. Hansen, Copley News Service, was published in the *Fayetteville Observer-Times* 10 June 1994, 3D.

[15]Howe, 120.

[16]Sharon R. Curtin, *Nobody Ever Died of Old Age* (Boston: Little, Brown, & Co., 1972) 50.

[17]Hutchison, 83.

[18]Arnold Toynbee, source unknown.

[19]Robert Browning, "Rabbi Ben Ezra," in *The Complete Poetic and Dramatic Works of Robert Browning*, ed. Horace E. Scudder (Boston: Houghton Mifflin 1898) 383.

[20]Howe, 161.

Death

Those in the fiery furnace find One who walks with them. Those who walk through the valley of the shadow of death do not walk alone. God, the Parent who so loved the world, became a co-sufferer with all parents who share Mount Moriah's supreme test of faith, through the gift and death of his beloved Son. . . .

At least when we challenge God, we keep a conversation going. That type of conversation is called prayer. And occasionally in the conversation, God interrupts, so to speak, and gets a word or two in edgewise. To hearts untroubled and hearts unsure, there is a window to heaven in the abiding promise that Jesus will come.

Diane M. Komp
A Window to Heaven[1]

Survivors of traumatic deaths suffer a uniquely wrenching loss that starts with shock and may end in familial and personal dysfunction. Along the way there are emotional challenges that cannot be avoided: disruption of family functioning; redefining responsibilities and roles of individual family members; challenges to faith; indifference or short-lived support from institutions previously depended on; financial change and burdens; possible intrusions by media (private anguish too often becomes a kaleidoscope for public voyeurism) and words and actions by friends and family that, often inadvertently, hurt.

Kenneth J. Doak
Living with Grief after Sudden Loss[2]

Death seems to have many faces and wears many masks. It disguises itself in numerous forms and meets us sometimes when we least expect it. Death is a universal experience; no one escapes it. An unseen virus can destroy the life of a robust athlete, and sometimes no one can prevent it nor understand its hidden path. A section of a train track is broken that causes a train to be derailed and hundreds of people are killed. Malfunctioning brakes cause the car a young couple is driving to crash head-on into a tractor trailer truck, and their lives are lost. A bolt that was manufactured improperly breaks, and one of the engines of an airplane falls off; the plane crashes, and hundreds of lives are lost. A tornado cuts a path through a community leaving behind devastation and havoc. A volcano tears an ugly hole in the earth and pours its fiery vapor upon all who are nearby, bringing death and destruction with its hot breath. "Why?" comes the cry.

I stood in the room of a fourteen-year-old girl, who for months had been dying with cancer. Doctors had amputated her leg earlier. She knew she was close to the end. She died much too soon and too young. "Why?" her parents asked.

I sat by the bed of a man who was very elderly. His mind had been gone for years, but his body lingered on—and so did the cost. The burden crushed down heavily upon the family. The jubilant comic, Grady Nutt, who could communicate the gospel effectively, lost his life in what seemed a needless accident. A young minister friend and his wife lost their first child a few hours after he was born. A note from a grandfather asked the question on everyone's mind—"Why?" A minister's wife died after struggling against cancer for months, leaving three children and a grieving husband.

The Shadow of Death

Death stalks us daily. It is a reality we cannot ignore. Many of you have walked through the dark valley of grief and have witnessed the shadow of death. Death seems such a scandal, a paradox, an enigma. We really do not know how to handle its presence or how to face its grim face, and so many of us simply spend our lives fleeing from it or trying to ignore it. The silence of God in these dark moments is a great test of our faith.

I met a young woman as I was walking across a college campus a number of years ago. She stopped me and said, "My friends ask me, 'How is your mother doing?' " Her mother had been quite ill. "And when I tell them that she is dead, they do not know what to say. They become very uncomfortable and finally just walk away." Those students, like most other people, were uneasy with the conversation focusing on death, and so they avoided it.

Have you noticed how most people react to the death of others or to the possibility of their own deaths? Almost everyone tries to deny the reality of death. Some denial takes the radical form of the Christian Science position of Mary Baker Eddy and asserts, "If sin, sickness, and death were understood as nothingness, they would disappear."[3] But sin, sickness, and death are not illusions. They are real.

The Reality of Death

Sin is a reality. I know it is real because I have sinned and have witnessed the sinfulness of others. We are all sinners. We also know that sickness is a reality. All of us at some time have been sick or have suffered. We know death is a reality because we have seen loved ones and friends who have been separated from us by it. When the wave of death sweeps over us, we cannot deny its presence. We may try to avoid it or deny it, but its reality will not evade us forever.

In one of the scenes in Noel Coward's play, *This Happy Breed*, Frank is talking to his sister, Sylvia, who has recently become a Christian Scientist. Frank's wife Ethel is back in the kitchen. Sylvia speaks, "There's not so much to do since Mrs. Flint passed on." Frank turns sharply and replies, "I do wish you wouldn't talk like that, Sylvia. It sounds so soft." "I don't know what you mean, I am sure," says Sylvia. "Mother died, see. First she got the flu, and that turned into pneumonia, and that affected the heart which was none too strong at the best of times, and she DIED! Nothing to do with passing on at all." "How do you know?" Sylvia responds. "I admit," Frank continues, "it's only your new way of talking, but it gets me down, see?" Then Ethel comes into the room and asks, "What are you shouting about?" "I'm not shouting about anything at all," Frank replies. "I'm merely explaining to Sylvia that Mother died! She didn't pass on or pass over or pass out—she DIED!"[4]

Death is a reality we must acknowledge, admit, and face. Most of us have difficulty even in verbalizing the words, "She died." We use euphemisms for death such as "expire," "gone away," "terminal illness," "gone on a long journey," or "gone to sleep." Others seek to disguise death. Funeral directors are experts at this. We pay the professionals to disguise the body of our loved ones so they do not appear to be dead, though of course, they are. We camouflage their death cosmetically to make them appear "natural."

A friend of mine, who had a conference on death and dying in his church, wrote an article in the church bulletin in which he observed, "I know this whole series has made many of you very uncomfortable, and I could sense that you have been uneasy. But it is ok, because we will be through it soon." But the question about death does not end when a series of sermons is concluded. The questions linger, because death and grief are realities with which we struggle all of our lives. This question cannot always be evaded or ignored.

An Attitude of Fate

Others approach death with an attitude of fate. Whatever is going to be will be. "When my time comes I will die," the man remarks. "I'm not going to die," the young soldier says, "until a bullet has my name on it." Where did he learn that philosophy of predeterminism or pre-destination? Those who live by this view sometimes take foolish chances, or do crazy things, assuming all the time that something or someone is going to protect them until their moment comes.

There is an ancient legend about a young man who rushed in to see the sultan in the city of Damascus. He told the sultan that he needed to borrow a horse and flee immediately to Baghdad. When the sultan asked him why he had to leave in such a hurry, he answered, "Because I was just going through the garden and I met Death. He stretched out his arms as if to seize me, and so I must lose no time escaping him." The sultan told him to take his own horse and leave at once for Baghdad. After he left, the sultan went down into his garden and found Death still there. "How dare you threaten one of my favorites?" the sultan demanded. "But your Majesty, I didn't threaten him at all," Death replied. "When I saw him, I just threw up my hands in surprise at seeing him here, because, you see, I have an appointment with him tonight in Baghdad."

In this approach to life, fate alone determines our destiny. "I'll go when my time comes," they declare, "and not a minute before." "If I'm in the right place at the right moment, then and only then will I die." These persons live out their lives in a kind of predeterminism that whatever is supposed to happen will come about and there is nothing anyone can do to change it or guide it.

The Atheistic Answer

Others live with an atheistic attitude and declare that the presence of death in the world is such a scandal that it removes all meaning from life. "How can there be a good God who is endless and eternal and, then, create humanity who dies? What kind of a God would make

that sort of world?" they ask. They shake their fist in the air and rage
against heaven and assert that death proves there is no God and there
could not be one. This kind of approach is reflected in many of the
contemporary short stories and novels of writers such as Camus,
Hemingway, Kafka, Sartre, and Beckett.

Ernest Hemingway, in a short story entitled, "A Clean, Well-
Lighted Place," wrote about an old man who would come into a bar
every night to drink. He would drink until closing time and, then, go
out and be swallowed up in the darkness of the night. His own empti-
ness was reflected by the parodying of the Hail Mary as, "Hail Nada,
full of Nada," and the Lord's Prayer as, "Our Nada which are in Nada,
Nada is thy name."[5] Nada is the Spanish word for "nothing." The old
man was on his own. He symbolized a kind of dignified atheism that
reflected his own ability to transcend his world to a degree but, nevertheless, he represents what it is like to live in a universe where there is
no God who transcends us. To use Amos Wilder's image, many now
live with a "secular transcendence."[6] Nothingness is all that one is left
to face when death comes. Death, then, is the ultimate scandal, the
dark enigma.

Death Seen as Natural

Most people fall in the category of viewing death as simply a natural
event. It is a biological happening, a part of the rhythm of nature.
Like the rest of nature, we come into being, exist a while, and then
perish. Nature consists of devouring and being devoured. Death is a
part of the total biological process of the cycle of life. All things that
come into existence, one day will die. Just as a dog dies, so we human
beings die. We are just biological creatures, and when our functions
wear out, we die. It is all very natural.

The New Testament concept does not view death merely as a biological matter. To some people, this biblical view is really more radical
than they realize. The apostle Paul, writing in his Roman epistle,
clearly states that death for the Christian is not just a part of a natural
occurrence. He declares that death has come about as a result of sin.

> It was through one man that sin entered the world, and through sin
> death, and thus death pervaded the whole human race, inasmuch as
> all have sinned. . . . But death held sway from Adam to Moses, even
> over those who had not sinned as Adam did by disobeying a direct
> command. (5:12-14 NEB)

Paul traces the origin of death to Adam. By the sin of Adam all persons have become sinners and separated from fellowship with God. Death is a consequence of sin. Through the righteousness of Christ, the new Adam, our broken relationship with God has been restored. Paul expresses this more clearly in another one of his letters.

> For since death came through a human being, the resurrection of the dead has also come through a human being; for as all die in Adam, so all will be made alive in Christ. (1 Cor 15:21-22)

Our Link with Others

In the Jewish mind, a person always saw one's self not merely as an individual but as a part of a family, tribe, or nation. One existed in solidarity with others. We are linked in solidarity with Adam. Adam was recognized as more than just a man who existed in the past and sinned; every one of us in our solidarity with Adam has actually sinned in Adam. Each of us sins, which reveals our Adam-like nature, but more than that our humanity binds us in the chain of being. In our solidarity with Adam, we, too, are also sinners.

Paul Achtemeier notes that the apostle Paul joined the figures of Adam and Christ to the two possible fates of humanity: sin, which leads to death, and grace, which leads to life. He continues,

> The problem of physical death as the result of sin is a major problem in the passage for the modern person. The reason lies in the fact that we are simply not accustomed to thinking of sin as a power capable of altering the structure of reality. . . . For Paul, those efforts reach all the way to an adverse effect on the very structure of reality.[7]

Paul's sense of the seriousness of sin shows why he felt it took the death of God's Son to overcome these effects. Only a radical event could restore such a serious break in the relationship between God and creation.

Sometimes we forget that each of us is Adam. I think John Whale expressed it well when he wrote:

> Eden is on no map, and Adam's fall fits no historical calendar. . . . The fall refers not to some datable aboriginal calamity in the historic past of humanity, but to a dimension of human experience

which is always present—namely, that we who have been created for fellowship with God repudiated it continually; and that the whole of mankind does this along with us. Every man is his own "Adam," and all men are solidarity "Adam."[8]

This theologian reminds us that just as Adam sinned so you and I continue to sin. Death is a reality that continues to attest to our sinful nature. By breaking a direct command of God, Adam suffered the consequences of his sin—which was death. Christ, in perfect obedience to God, has overcome the power of sin and brought newness of life and has conquered the power of death. Adam—humankind—was created for fellowship with God, but this fellowship was broken by sin. Since sin had separated humanity from God, men and women have continued to long again for this communion with God. Through Christ this communion once again was established. Christ is the new Adam. He is the one who restores the broken relationship that was severed between God and the human family. He has brought us back together in fellowship with God.

It has always been interesting to me that one of the favorite hymns that is often selected at funerals is "Nearer, My God to Thee." Death is not viewed as a natural process in which persons are separated further from God, but hymns like this symbolize the yearning to draw closer to God even in death. Through Christ, the chasm of death has been overcome, and we are brought closer into a vital relationship with God. Death, from the Christian perspective, is not just a biological event. It is a contradiction in the relationship that was originally established to exist between God and humankind. Death has left us with a sense of incompleteness that is only resolved in the redemptive work of Christ. Whether we can fully grasp it or not, the New Testament declares that death came into the world as a result of sin and is not simply a biological happening.

The Illusion of Immortality

We all still like to live with the illusion that we are immortal, don't we? None of us wants to face the fact that one day we will die. Nobody wants to see the sign on the meter of life that reads, "Time expired." We feel like we can continue to put some kind of quarters in life's parking meter, and our time will go on endlessly. But we need to realize that life does have a point of termination. A part of our illusion about life is that, like Adam, we want to be Superman. We assert that we are Prometheus. We want to be free of limitations or controls. We do not want to be bound by our humanity. We want to be above God. We long to be a god. We think we can control God. Like Adam, we reach for the forbidden fruit and eat it so that we can have the knowledge and eternity of God. But that is our basic sin, isn't it? What an illusion we cling to in our thinking that we can be like God and have no sin to confess!

The illusion of immortality clings to us. We refuse immediately to face the fact of our own death. In his Pulitzer Prize winning book entitled *The Denial of Death,* Ernest Becker says that death

> haunts the human animal like nothing else; it is a mainspring of human activityæactivity designed largely to avoid the fatality of death, to overcome it by denying in some way that it is the final destiny for man.[9]

We continuously deny our mortality, but none of us evades death. The word death is like a four-letter word that has been forbidden to be uttered. To mention the word death is like one daring to use the ultimate word of profanity. We do everything to avoid its use and to deny its reality. We repress, disguise, deny, ignore, or belie our fear of death and cling to the illusion that we shall never die.

George Papashuily grew up in Caucasus, Russia. In his town, it was the custom for all of the young boys to visit a hermit who lived in the mountains. A young boy customarily took a small gift when he went to see the hermit, and in exchange, the hermit would give him a proverb. The hermit motioned to him, and he went over to the revered old man. After asking him several questions, he whispered into his ear, "This minute, too, is a part of eternity." Papashuily said that it was a long time before he was able to grasp the meaning of that saying. Later he would come to realize that birth, death, and all of life in between are parts of a harmonious whole.

Life as a Gift from God

Reject the illusion of immortality and realize that the minute you have today is a gift from God. "This is the day that the Lord has made; let us rejoice and be glad in it" (Ps 118:24). Utilize this moment, this hour, this day, this week, this year because no one of us knows how many moments, days, or years we may have. Each minute comes to us as a gift from God. Just suppose that you thought or knew that you were going to die at the end of this year. Would you live your life differently? Would you reorder it in any way? What would be your priorities? What would be the items at the top of your agenda for living? What would be most important? How would you seek to live to the fullest the time you have?

Remember, each of us has only a limited time span. What will you do with the gift of the time you have? Suppose death did not exist. When would we ever get around to start living? Death rather than being the great scandal that removes all meaning gives us the limits that make life meaningful. The awareness of death forces us to learn to live within a limited time frame, to take time seriously, to take ourselves seriously, to take relationships seriously, and to take the responsibility of getting on with living seriously.

With the acknowledgment of death, we confirm our awareness of our limited existence; therefore, we seek to grasp time, use time, spend time wisely—not carelessly or foolishly—but to invest it into all we do so that we can reap meaningfulness and worthwhileness from all the time we live. Death is not the destroyer of meaning; it is the partition—the fence—that gives us the limits of our own existence as we seek to live out our years with purpose and direction.

Stages in Dying

One of the classic studies on what the dying can teach the living is Elizabeth Kubler-Ross's work *On Death and Dying*. In her pioneering work, Dr. Kubler-Ross studied terminally ill patients and their responses to death and what the living could do to assist them. She observed five basic stages persons usually go through in their process of dying.

The first stage of dying is denial. Most people simply cannot believe that they are dying. They think that it has to be a mistake. They assume that the doctor must have made a mistake, and so they look to another source for help. Denial is the first reaction.

The second stage a person enters may be one of anger. A terminal person's anger is sometimes directed at the doctor or one's husband or wife, or the nurses, or the minister, or at anyone who happens to come by. Sometimes the person may direct her anger even at God. As relatives or friends or as the dying person, we need to learn that it is ok to be angry. It is all right even to be angry with God. God will accept our anger and still love us. Let us acknowledge to our friends and relatives that anger is a normal part of the process of dying.

A third stage of dying often finds a person attempting to bargain with relatives, friends, doctors, or even God. "God," they say, "if you will let me live until my son graduates from high school or until June is married or this special event, I promise to . . ."

The next stage is usually depression, and, then, finally acceptance. Everyone does not go through all of these stages, but an awareness of the normal stages of death can help us relate to those who are dying.

I remember a couple with whom I had the privilege of ministering during the months the husband was dying from cancer. Over a period of several months, I saw them grow in their ability to communicate with each other and discuss openly the fact that he was dying. The last months of their lives were some of the most marvelous experiences they had ever had. It came about because of their openness to each other and their willingness to share their inner feelings. On several occasions they went back to the place where they first met and the little park where they used to go on dates when they were young. They talked endlessly, made preparations to sell his business, drew up a will, and attempted to settle all the loose ends before he died. He spent time with his children and grandchildren.

Few have the opportunity to make all of those kinds of preparations, because many people die suddenly. But when there is opportunity, let communication take place between you and your loved one or friend who is dying. Sometimes just knowing the normal stages people go through when they are dying will enable us to be more responsive and helpful.

Ways to Help the Dying

When persons are dying, they have fears and longings in this part of life's journey. The following are some positive suggestions on ways you might strengthen a friend or family member as they confront their own mortality.

Do Not Isolate Them

When you have a friend or relative who is dying, try to help the person from feeling isolated. "There is almost nothing as crushing to a dying patient as to feel that he has been abandoned or rejected." "The sting of death is solitude," states Paul Ramsey. "Desertion is more choking than death and more feared."[10] A great fear of many people who are dying is that they will be cut off and isolated from family and friends. They fear that no one will come to see them and they will be deserted. They do not want to be separated from friends and loved ones. Even if they are in the hospital or in ICU, continue to sustain them with your visit.

Most people prefer to die at home among their friends rather than at a hospital. I am convinced that one of the reasons for this is their desire not to be left alone. A woman told me about the satisfaction of having her father die in her arms. He had been ill for months and they debated about going to the hospital in the final days, but decided against it and were pleased later by the time they had been able to share together. Some people, of course, should be in the hospital to receive the kind of help they need. Others should not. When someone is like the person whose world is confined to the four corners of the bed, then other assistance may be needed. But even then, continue to sustain them with your visits.

Encourage Them to Express Their Feelings

Remember to let the dying express their feelings. Don't tell them, "Oh, don't talk to me about your feelings or fears. I don't want to hear it." They really want to talk to someone. Most dying people long to share their feelings with their loved ones and selected friends. Let them express their fears, hopes, pain, or longings. Listen to them, and even encourage them to talk. Be a willing ear. Do not turn away from them when they long for someone to whom they can express their feelings. You can be a sounding board for their bottled up emotions. Remember the various stages they may be going through and permit them to be honest and to express their feelings.

Touch Them

Remember to continue to touch the dying. Ashley Montagu observed that "touch is the mother of all sense."[11] Touch is probably the first sense a baby has, and touch is likely the last sensation dying people have. Hold their hand, kiss them, embrace them, massage them. Let them feel your presence through touch. Remember that our Lord continued to reach out his hand and touched the "untouchables"—the leper, the blind, the lame, the outcasts, sinners, the beggar, children, women, the sick, and many others. He touched all who had a need. Continue to give the dying your presence, your care and concern, the assurance of your support.

Maintain a Positive Attitude

Also remember to maintain a positive approach with the dying regarding their illness. Give them some element of encouragement, even if there appears to be little hope. Your attitude and treatment of them should not take away all hope. Do not give them over to death too quickly. Norman Cousins wrote about the difference this positive emphasis could make.

> If negative emotions produce negative chemical changes in the body, wouldn't the positive emotions produce positive chemical changes? Is it possible that love, hope, faith, laughter, confidence, and the will to live have therapeutic values?[12]

He discovered that, of course, they could. William James said, "Human beings tend to live too far within self-imposed limits."[13] Do not cut the terminally ill persons off from all hope—even if it is hope for less pain, more time with the family, or the presence of a concerned friend. Try to communicate messages of hope and encouragement in all that you do for them.

Affirm Our Trust in God

Even when we are aware of the reality of death around us, we ultimately have to live out our lives in trust. No one has an easy or final answer to the whole question of death and the enigma of suffering and pain. But as Christians, we still trust God. We affirm our trust in the God who is "from everlasting to everlasting." Paul testified to his own faith when he declared:

> If we live, we live for the Lord; and if we die, we die for the Lord. Whether therefore we live or die, we belong to the Lord. This is why Christ died and came to life again, to establish his lordship over dead and living. (Rom 14:7-9 NEB)

Easter is the Christian celebration of the reality of life out of death that we experience through Jesus Christ our Lord. The last enemy to be destroyed, Paul said, is death. The power of death is overcome in Christ.

Nicholas Wolterstorff's world was shattered when he received
word that his twenty-five-year-old son, Eric, had been killed in a
mountain climbing accident in Austria. As this Christian philosopher
struggled with the "why" of such an event, he came up with no easy
answer. He acknowledged that some suffering and death could be the
result of sin caused by war, assault, poverty in the midst of plenty, and
so on. He realized that some suffering could be the result of chastisement, but not all. He concluded,

> The meaning of the remainder is not told us. It eludes us. Our net
> of meaning is too small. There's more to our suffering than our
> guilt. A religion that does not affirm that God is hidden is not true.
> . . . God reveals Himself. He speaks, yes. But as he speaks, he hides.
> His face he does not show us.

Out of his pain, Wolterstorff still affirmed, "Faith is a footbridge that
you don't know will hold you up over the chasm until you're forced to
walk out onto it."[14]

On December 21, 1962, L. D. Johnson received word that his
young daughter, Carole, who had celebrated her twenty-third birthday
the day before, had been killed in a tragic automobile accident. She
had graduated earlier from the University of Richmond, received a
master's degree from the University of North Carolina, and had taught
high school for only one semester. She was driving home to Green-
ville, South Carolina, for the Christmas holidays when her small
compact car collided with a tractor-trailer truck. Her life had been
filled with joy and excitement, and she was to have been married
shortly. For sixteen years Dr. Johnson could not write about his experience, but several years ago he published a book entitled *The Morning
After Death* in which he wrote about Carole's death.

He did not try to give an explanation for her death. He acknowledged that she lost her life in a senseless, meaningless tragedy for
which he could not find a good purpose. "The mystery of unmerited
suffering remains. I know of no satisfactory explanation. But for the
Christian there is an answer—not an explanation."[15] He found that
there is no simple answer to suffering and death, but there is trust in
the Answerer. We still trust in God. We do not know why tragic accidents happen. We cannot explain the how of them, but that does not
mean we cannot rely upon the presence of God to sustain us. In his
worst kind of grief and tragedy, Dr. Johnson affirmed that God's

presence was with him. He didn't know the why of the accident, and he deeply regretted that this young life would never be able to fulfill all of its potential, but he still knew that God was good. He trusted God though he had no answer. He continued to lean heavily upon the one who was the answerer—God.

Death will come into all of our lives—sometimes quietly or screaming—but, when it comes, we need not run in fear from it, but we, like the apostle Paul, can place our trust in the God who has been with us in life and will be with us in death. The God who has sustained us in life will sustain us in death. United with Christ, we live out our lives in trust, knowing that God will bear us safely through our vale of tears.

Notes

[1]Diane M. Komp, *A Window to Heaven* (Grand Rapids: Zondervan, 1992) 120.

[2]Kenneth J. Doak, ed., *Living with Grief after Sudden Loss* (Bristol PA: Taylor & Francis, 1996) 17.

[3]Mary Baker Eddy, *Science and Health with Key to the Scriptures*, published by trustees under the will of Mary Baker Eddy (Boston, 1934) 107.

[4]Noel Coward, *This Happy Breed* (Garden City NY: Doubleday, 1947) 178.

[5]Ernest Hemingway, "A Clean, Well-Lighted Place," in *Winner Take Nothing* (New York: Charles Scribner's Sons, 1933) 23.

[6]Amos Wilder, "Mortality and Contemporary Literature," in *The Modern Version of Death*, ed Nathan A. Scott, Jr. (Richmond VA: John Knox Press, 1967) 25f.

[7]Paul Achtemeier, *Romans, Interpretation: A Bible Commentary for Teaching and Preaching* (Atlanta: John Knox Press, 1985) 99.

[8]John Whale, *Christian Doctrine* (London: Fontana Books, 1958) 49.

[9]Ernest Becker, *The Denial of Death* (New York: Free Press, 1975) ix.

[10] Paul Ramsey, *The Meaning of Death,* Herman Feifel, ed. (New York: McGraw-Hill, 1959) 125.

[11]Ashley Montagu, *Touching: The Human Significance of Skin* (New York: Harper & Row, 1971) 1.

[12]Norman Cousins, *Anatomy of an Illness* (New York: W. W. Norton, 1979) 34-35.

[13]Ibid, 48.

[14]Nicholas Wolerstorff, *Lament for a Son* (Grand Rapids: Eerdmans, 1987) 74-76.

[15]L. D. Johnson, *The Morning After Death* (Macon GA: Smyth & Helwys, 1995) 113.

Light Out of Darkness

The argument is unanswerable; and is indeed the only unanswerable argument for immortality that has ever been given, or ever can be given. It cannot be evaded except by a denial of the premises. If the individual can commune with God, then he must matter to God; and if he matters to God, he must share God's eternity. For if God really rules, He cannot be conceived as scrapping what is precious in His sight. It is in the conjunction with God that the promise of eternal life resides.

John Baillie
And the Life Everlasting[1]

The historical fact that the resurrection of the dead was solidified into a doctrine of Judaism not until a relatively late time explains also its rationality. Unlike the mystery cults of Egypt, Greece, and Asia Minor, which also believed in the resurrection, it is free from magic, mysticism, miraculousness, and lengthy burial rites, which often degenerated into worship of the dead.

If God is all-just and all-merciful, then death in this world cannot be the final end.

Pinchas Lapide
The Resurrection of Jesus
A Jewish Perspective[2]

It is time, therefore, for the remnants of classical Christianity on this continent to counter all the rumors of a catastrophic ending that emanate from either religious or secular sources by professing their faith in a God who wills to complete and fulfill the promises of a creation that has been visited and redeemed by the love that made it.

Douglas John Hall
Professing the Faith[3]

Several decades ago, Clarence Hall, the late editor of *Reader's Digest*, went to Israel for an Easter sunrise service of worship. He was unable to sleep, and the night grew long for him. He became quarrelsome with his Christian Arab guide and asked him if the night would ever end so he could go to the Garden Tomb for the service. "Never fear, my friend," Abdul, his guide responded. "The day will come. You can't hold back the dawn."

The Reality of Darkness

When Christians declare that Jesus Christ is alive, this does not mean that there is no darkness in the world. Darkness continues to exist, and we acknowledge its presence quickly and readily. During the Second World War, more than six million Jews were put to death. That darkness was deep with despair. Terrorism sticks its ugly head all around the world today. The wars that have flared up around the globe and others that continue to erupt here and there indicate something about the darkness that prevails in the world. You and I know something about our own personal darkness as well. I have walked with many persons to a graveside to bury a loved one. I have sat by a hospital bed with those who have seen a life dear to them slip away. The edge of darkness has touched us all.

A wife telephoned her husband at lunch time. She was to meet him in a few minutes, and they were going out for lunch. But when she arrived at his office moments later, he was dead. Before she arrived, he had died from a cerebral hemorrhage. She then began to walk into the dark valley of grief.

A young couple sat in the hospital with their two-year-child who was dying with cancer. Their agony was so apparent, and the child was so young. He was just beginning his life, and they feared that it soon might end. A dark cloud hung over them.

The former mayor of a large city and his mother were killed in an automobile accident. A local paper told about a couple who was robbed and murdered in their home. The same paper carried a report about a young woman who had been married only a year and was raped by an escaped convict. Thousands die from starvation in Africa. There is darkness around us in many places in the world today. Its face is visible in the problems of drugs, alcoholism, war, famine, AIDS, disease, and poverty. Many are trapped in their darkness and are not able to find light out of that darkness.

No one can deny that darkness is in the world. The writer of the Gospel of John declares clearly and without apology in his prologue (1:1-5) that, although there is darkness in the world, the darkness has not mastered the light that has been revealed in Jesus Christ. John recognized the darkness of evil, ignorance, sin, suffering, and death. John contrasted light and darkness. The darkness had not overcome the light. As Christians we continue to affirm that Jesus Christ is alive and at work in the world. Darkness has not won. His light is still visible.

The Light of Easter

It was a dark night two thousand years ago when the disciples gathered together in an upper room. They were hiding from the religious authorities, fearful that they themselves would be put to death like their Lord. They were huddled together, frightened, filled with despair, hopeless in the face of what had happened. Friday began their long trip into the pit of darkness.

On Sunday morning a group of women approached the tomb of Jesus to anoint his body. They had not been able to place aromatic spices on his body since he was crucified and died just as the Sabbath was beginning. The Sabbath was not over, and on Sunday morning they approached the tomb. They wondered how they would roll away the stone. Graves in biblical times were often built in a mountainside. A huge groove was chiseled out in front of the tomb, and a flat stone about the size of an ox-wheel was placed in the groove and rolled in front of the entrance to the tomb. Sometimes it took two men to roll the stone away so that one could get into the grave. "Who would roll away the stone?" they wondered. When they arrived at the tomb, however, they found that the stone had already been rolled away and that Jesus Christ had risen from the grave.

In the light of Easter Sunday morning, reflect on the power that raised Jesus Christ from the grave, and the power his spirit has today in our lives to roll back the stones that keep us within tombs of deadness and despondency. Christ meets us today to offer us his aliveness. Easter reminds us again that the Lord of life is still with us today. The entry to our lives is often blocked with stones that prevent us from being alive to the presence and power of God. We are inhibited because the doorway of our life is blocked. We need the power of God to roll away the stone.

Jesus has promised to provide the way for us. "I am the gate; whoever enters by me will be saved, and will come in and go out and find pasture" (John 10:9). "Listen! I am standing at the door, knocking; if you hear my voice and open the door, I will come in to you and eat with you, and you with me" (Rev 3:20). When the entrance of our life is opened to the presence of Christ, we enjoy his fellowship and the redeeming power he brings into our innermost being. Jesus is constantly rolling away stones that block our lives and removing barriers that prevent us from sharing in real life.

In the story of the raising of Lazarus from his tomb in Bethany, Jesus said to Martha, "I am the resurrection and the life. Those who believe in me, even though they die, will live, and everyone who lives and believes in me will never die" (John 11:25). He asked that the stone be removed from the tomb of Lazarus. Then he cried with a loud voice, "Lazarus, come out." Lazarus came out of the tomb, and Jesus told those around him, "Unbind him, and let him go." As the living Lord, he comes into your dead life and mine and sets us free from our tombs. He unbinds us and sets us free to live.

The Unauthentic Life

One of the stones Jesus rolls back that blocks our lives and buries us within tombs is the stone of the unauthentic life. Many of us live out our lives in an artificial way. We have never really experienced authentic life. Jesus said that "I came that they may have life, and have it abundantly" (John 10:10). Some of us have never experienced the abundant life. The quality of life Christ came to give is missing from the lives of many. "I am the resurrection and the life" (John 11:25), he declared. His life is a present possession.

Several years ago in Texas, a millionaire was being buried. As they sometimes do things in Texas, this man's funeral was conducted in a rather extravagant way. He was being buried in his gold Cadillac. He was placed in his car in a position sitting up behind the steering wheel, wearing a white suit and a white hat, and with a cigar in his mouth. As they were lowering his car into the grave, somebody said, "Man, that's living!" But it was not; it was death.

Some people continue to confuse life and death. Many have not been able to see the distinction between the inferior life—a life wrapped up in material ends—and the life we have in Jesus Christ. In his gospel, John used the word "life" thirty-five times and the words "to live" fifteen times. He stressed the difference Christ made in a person's life. Christ has come that we may have life and have it with abundant meaning.

A number of years ago Ingmar Bergman produced a movie entitled *Wild Strawberries*. In this movie a professor dreamed that he was taking his morning walk. In his dream, he saw a funeral procession and a wagon carrying a coffin. As the wagon turned a corner and entered the churchyard, the coffin fell off the wagon. The corpse was thrown out of the coffin and landed at his feet. The professor reluctantly took hold of the body to put it back in the coffin. But a strange thing happened when he touched the body. The corpse grabbed his arm, and they struggled for a few moments until they were face to face. As the professor looked into the face of the dead man, in horror he saw himself. When he awoke from his dream, he knew instantly what the dream meant. He knew he had been living and acting as though he were a dead man. He was a walking corpse. It was a terrible dream, but it changed his life.

Many of us live in the world today as though we were dead persons. We have never experienced authentic life. We are only shadows of what God has created us to be, mere reflections of authentic life. The real, abundant, joyful life God has come to give us in Christ, we have not experienced. We live only on the edge of life. We have not felt life in its fullness, when the transforming presence of Christ is in our life. We only exist; we live as dead persons. Christ came to roll away the stone of inferior life and to give us real life. The eternal life Christ gives us begins now. "This is eternal life," John says, "that they may know you, the only true God, and Jesus Christ whom you have sent" (John 17:3). "In him was life; and the life was the light of all people" (John 1:4).

Human Frailty

Jesus Christ comes to the tomb of our lives and also rolls away the stone of human frailty. One of our struggles with life, of course, is our own sense of coming to grips with our humanity. We would like to deny our humanity and pretend that we are super persons and ignore our weak efforts to handle many problems. After the crucifixion of Jesus, the disciples huddled together in a hidden room, feeling powerless and frightened. The door was bolted shut against the religious authorities, and their weakness and cowardliness controlled them. Later, on Sunday morning, a group of women approached the tomb of Jesus to anoint his body, but they did not think they would be strong enough to move the stone that blocked his grave. Their limitations revealed their human frailty.

But you and I know something about our own frailty, don't we? You might have come to those moments in your life when your health has failed, or you have faced an operation and have felt keenly your own sense of frailty. A loved one of yours has had an illness or a heart attack or a stroke, and you huddle around them, feeling helpless in the situation. There are some who have felt your marriage pulled apart and your life wrenched by divorce. You felt helpless in this crisis and did not know what to do or where to turn. There are some who have been pulled down by drugs and feel their lives are out of control. Drink has driven some people almost to despair; they feel helpless. They long for someone or something to give them strength and direction. The apostle Paul asserted, "I can do all things through him who strengthens me" (Phil 4:13). Christ meets us in our frailty and offers us his strength and power. He comes as a living presence to sustain us and give us a resource we have not known.

When Robert Louis Stevenson was a young boy, one day he was playing in a cupboard at his home. He accidently locked himself inside and screamed for help. His father heard his call for help and tried to open the cupboard but could not. A repairman had to be sent for to open the cupboard. While they waited for the repairman to arrive, the father continued to talk to his young son who was trapped inside. Stevenson said that, although he was surrounded by darkness and the cupboard was filled with dust and cobwebs, he was comforted by the strength of his father whose presence sustained him by talking to him through the door until he was released.

God has not told us that all of the darkness, difficulties, or pain will be removed, but we have the assurance that God is present with us in all of these experiences. We can "hear" God's voice, feel the strength of the divine presence that empowers us to meet whatever difficulties we encounter. God rolls away the stone of our inadequacy, and God's living presence gives us strength to live with and beyond our humanity.

Skepticism

God also comes into our lives through the risen Christ to roll back the stone of disbelief. Jesus had told his disciples on numerous occasions that after his crucifixion, he would rise from the grave. We forget, however, that the disciples really did not believe that Christ would rise from the grave, as evidenced by their absence from the tomb site. If they had really believed that Jesus Christ would rise from the grave on Sunday morning, they would have stood there in troops—waiting, waiting, waiting for him to rise. But they did not believe it, and they were not there.

The women who came to the tomb on Sunday morning did not come to celebrate his resurrection; they came to anoint a dead body. They were startled, amazed, and terrified when they found that he was risen. Thomas expressed the view of many when he declared that "unless I see the mark of the nails in his hands, and put my finger in the mark of the nails and my hands in his side, I will not believe" (John 20:25). Thomas symbolizes our own questions, fears, and doubts about Christ.

Jesus Christ enters our world of disbelief and changes our doubts to faith and questions to answers. Too many find their faith tested by the advances of science and feel intimidated when someone has a question they are unable to answer. We are also threatened by the problems of pain, suffering, and evil in the world and do not know where to turn to solve them. Sometimes we are victims of our moods. Our attitude toward God is determined by whether we are tired, lonely, depressed, or ill. If our spirit is up, we can worship God, but when we are down, we can't. Our moods reflect our understanding of how we are supposed to relate to God. God becomes a victim of our moods.

But God is not limited by your moods or my moods. God is not at the mercy of our mood swings or emotional level. Christians need not fear scientific questions or the inability to answer them or their changing mood or the unsolvable problem of suffering and evil. The presence of Christ assures us of his guidance through the maze or struggle we will continually have with disbelief. Even when our faith is weak, or our convictions unsteady, or our hope insecure, or our offense grievous, we are confident of Christ's forgiveness, support, and presence.

Several years ago in Florida a religious play was performed at Easter entirely by the prisoners of the state penitentiary. The play made some modification in the gospel story about the life and death of Christ and had a scene in the play where Judas came back and fell down at the feet of Christ and asked for forgiveness. "Lord, have mercy on me. Forgive me," Judas cried. The prisoners were so moved by the scene that they would break into applause, and the play was so disrupted by their applause that the directors of the play finally erected a sign that stated, "No applause, please."

The prisoners may have grasped a deep religious truth. Though that play may not be exactly like the gospel record, I am convinced that if Judas had come back to our Lord and asked for forgiveness, Christ would have forgiven him. He forgave those who nailed him to the cross, and he would have forgiven Judas. When you are pulled down to despair by your questions of disbelief, or your doubts weight heavy on your mind, or your low mood makes you feel that God has withdrawn from you, be assured that God is near to you and strengthens you by God's living presence. God has rolled away the stone of disbelief and given us instead an open door to truth and assurance.

The Need for Forgiveness

There are also some today who need to have the stone of unforgiveness removed from the entrance of their lives. It is blocking them from authentic living. Many live with a nagging sense of guilt and pain for something they might have done in the past and have not yet experienced God's forgiveness, love, and grace. Judas and Peter both betrayed their Lord. After his betrayal, Judas, in despair, went out and hanged himself. He could not live with what he had done, and he had not found forgiveness. Simon Peter later met the risen Christ by the seashore, and Christ asked him if he loved him. Peter acknowledged he did, forgiveness was given, and restoration took place. Judas took the leap of despair, while Peter made a leap of faith.

There are some today who are still clinging to unforgiven sins, old guilts, and broken relationships. You have never heard the words of God: "You are forgiven." You are acceptable to God, because God is a God who loves you and will forgive you. Accept God's grace. Do not bury yourself in a tomb of unforgiven sins, guilt, misunderstandings, and despondency. God is a loving God who wants to forgive you.

Have you heard about barnacles? Barnacles are tiny sea creatures about the size of a walnut that attach themselves to the bottom of ships that sail the ocean. When they collect on the bottom of a ship over a period of months, they can sometimes add a hundred tons of weight to a single oceangoing liner and slow a huge ship's movement in the water by 10 percent. The only way to remove them is with a jackhammer while the ship is in dry dock.

Some of you today have a heavy load of "barnacles" of unconfessed, unforgiven sins, and guilt in your lives. You can experience forgiveness. When I talk with people in the hospitals, or in their homes, or in my study, I am amazed at how many people are carrying around with them heavy burdens of guilt and sins for which they have never yet experienced God's word of grace and love. Hear God's word today: "I forgive you. Start again." Accept your acceptance by God. God loves you and will forgive you.

Several years ago when I was in England, I visited the beautiful Coventry Cathedral outside London. After touring the cathedral, I walked out into the courtyard. Some of the charred remains of the earlier church, which had been bombed during the Second World War, were set up as a worship center in the courtyard. This garden was a reminder of the devastation the church had suffered earlier. A cross had been made from the charred remains of some timbers from the building, and written across the top of the cross were the words: "Father Forgive." The church community had asked forgiveness for their enemies.

In the worst kinds of circumstances you may experience, hear again the words that come to you from God when God says you are forgiven. Open yourself to God's redeeming grace that gives you another opportunity to begin your life again.

Hopelessness

The early disciples were also trapped behind the stone of cynicism and despair. After the death of Christ, some of the disciples felt like they might as well go back to their old jobs. There was nothing they could do now that Jesus was dead. Where could they turn? Christ had been crucified. Their dream of God's kingdom being established was over. It was hopeless. They gathered together in a dark room. They were filled with despair, and did not know what to do or where to go. Hopelessness, futility, and depression covered them with a dark cloud.

Some persons today live out their lives under this hopeless perspective. Their attitude is reflected in the old song, "Life gets tedious though, don't it?" In his humorous way, Jimmy Robertson used to sing about the hard times when the well and the cow go dry, the chickens quit laying, and he was getting dandruff, too. "Life gets tedious, don't it though?" he sang. For some, life does seem arduous and disquieting. They see no point to it and no direction. Sometimes a person will ask, "Is this all there is to it?" The words cry out with pain, frustration, and anger.

I recall talking with a young man who had hit the bottom of his life. He was suffering from deep depression and despair. After a long night, he turned and spoke to people the next morning as they passed him on the street. But he received no response from them. He began to wonder if he really existed. Was this a dream he was having? He decided to see if what he was experiencing was real or a dream. He walked into a store, got something from a shelf, took some money from his pocket, and walked over and gave the money to the clerk. "I knew I was real," he said, "when the clerk took my money." Some of us can slip into low pits of despair and need help to get out of them. There are some who are driven to the pits of despondency in their lives, and they grope for meaning, purpose, and hope in their life.

A young girl asked her father, after he had been rushing her to get into the car, "Daddy, when we get where we are going, where are we going to be?" When you get where you are rushing to go in your life—going day and night, hours without end to achieve your goal, acquiring so many things quickly and so fast—when you reach that goal, where will you be? Will you have real life when you get there, or will you end up only in despair? When you get where you are going in your work, marriage, family, free time, old age, where will you be? Will your life be filled with meaning? Christ's way guides us into the abundant life that seeks to fill all of our living with purpose and joy.

Overcoming Death

Easter assures us most of all that God has rolled back the stone of death and that we can have eternal life. The disciples did not really believe at first that they had found the life God had offered to them. Jesus Christ said earlier at the tomb of Lazarus, "I am the resurrection and the life. Those who believe in me . . . will never die" (John 11:25). But I am not sure that the disciples heard him then. That statement took on real meaning for them only after the resurrection.

The apostle Paul wrote in one of his epistles, "If Christ has not been raised, your faith is futile and you are still in your sins" (1 Cor 15:17). "Christianity stands or falls with the reality of the raising of Jesus Christ from the dead by God," the contemporary theologian Jurgen Moltmann declares. "In the New Testament there is no faith that does not start a priori from the resurrection."[4] Wolfhart Pannenberg, another contemporary theologian, affirms,

> In the resurrection of Jesus we therefore have to do with the sustaining foundation of the Christian faith. If this collapses, so does everything else which the Christian faith acknowledges.[5]

Without the resurrection there is no real authentic Christian faith. The resurrection is the foundation stone upon which our faith is built. The disciples had not expected the resurrection; they had not planned for it nor contemplated it. But when Christ arose from the grave, that group of disciples, who had given way to despair and pessimism, was transformed and went forth proclaiming fearlessly the good news. One of the strongest pieces of evidence for the resurrection of Christ is the existence of the Christian church. The church came into being because of the resurrection of Jesus Christ. After seeing the living Lord, the disciples were new persons filled with hope, courage, faith, and joy. They served a Lord who was alive! The power of the risen Christ changed them completely.

The Darkness Has Not Mastered the Light

There are some today who see only the power of darkness. Death is the final curtain of darkness that falls upon us. Some of us feel that life exists only for a moment. Like a lighted match that is extinguished quickly by the wind, our lives are over in a moment. The light of every life seems to ignite into a burst of flame ever so briefly and is soon gone. Does the darkness of death prevail? Has its shadow left such a black image on our life that all meaning has gone from living? If so, darkness would have mastered the light. But the Gospel of John assures us that the darkness has not overcome the light. His light continues to shine in the darkness (1:5).

One night on the Johnny Carson show a Hollywood starlet spoke about being deeply religious. Johnny asked her, "What do you believe?" "Oh, I don't believe anything in particular," she responded. "But I am deeply religious." I want to affirm loudly and clearly that the Christian gospel has to do with believing something in particular. It begins with the strong affirmation that Jesus Christ is alive. Our faith is built on the reality of his aliveness. His resurrection is the foundation of our faith. Because he lives, we shall live also.

My wife likes to read historical biographies, and a number of years ago she shared some sections with me from one she was reading on Patrick Henry. In 1799, Patrick Henry delivered a speech at the Charlotte courthouse. He returned home shortly after speaking and wrote a letter to President Adams declining to accept an appointment as ambassador to France. For some months he had felt quite ill. Dr. Cabble, who had been his physician through the years, knew that he was suffering from intussusception, an acute inflammation of the intestines. (Today that condition could be treated.)

Dr. Cabble walked into his old friend's bedroom and told him that he wanted to make a desperate attempt to see if he could help his condition. He wanted him to drink a vial of liquid mercury to see if it would help. "What will be the effect of this medicine?" Henry asked. "It will give you immediate relief," Dr. Cabble said, "or . . ." And he could not finish. "You mean, doctor," Henry responded, "that it will give relief or prove fatal immediately." "You can only live a very short time without it," the doctor replied. "And it may possibly relieve you." Henry pulled his silk nightcap down over his eyes and offered a simple prayer that one of his grandsons recorded. He prayed for his country, for his family, and for his own soul as he faced death. Then he took the vial of mercury and drank it.

Dr. Cabble went out into the yard and fell on the ground under some trees and wept bitterly. In a few moments he returned and noticed that the blood was beginning to congeal under Henry's fingernails, and knew that death was coming soon. Patrick Henry called his children over one by one and spoke with them. Then he called his old friend the doctor over. They had had many debates about the Christian faith. He expressed praise for his religion and asked the doctor to look upon a man whose faith had not failed him in all of his life, and, then he asked Dr. Cabble "to observe how great a reality and benefit that religion was to a man about to die."[6]

Later this man, who had served five times as governor of Virginia, was buried in a simple grave at Red Hill, Virginia. In his will were these words of testimony to his faith: "This is all the inheritance I give to my dear family. The religion of Christ can give them one which will make them rich indeed."[7] That is an affirmation each of us as Christians should be able to make. The stone of death has been rolled back in Jesus Christ who is alive today. To know the Son is to share eternal life.

Stones have trapped many of us in all kinds of tombs. Some are imprisoned in tombs of jealousy, selfishness, envy, despair, and pessimism. Centuries ago, Jesus stood in Bethany before the grave of Lazarus and cried to him, "Come forth." And he did! Christ stands before you today and speaks directly to those who are trapped in tombs. In a loud voice he cries to you, "Come forth." The living Christ is still striving to free us from the tombs that keep us from experiencing real life. He calls to let us know that we can have life and have it abundantly. He calls us out of darkness into light. One of the writers of the ancient psalms expressed his distress and then assurance of God in these powerful lines:

> I cried aloud to God, I cried to God, and he heard me. In the day of my distress I sought the Lord, and by night I lifted my outspread hands in prayer. I lay sweating and nothing would cool me; I refused all comfort. When I called God to mind, I groaned; as I lay thinking, darkness came over my spirit. My eyelids were tightly closed; I was dazed and I could not speak. My thoughts went back to times long past, I remembered forgotten years; all night long I was in deep distress, as I lay thinking, my spirit was sunk in despair. Will the Lord reject us for evermore and never again show favour? Has his unfailing love now failed us utterly, must his promise time and again be unfulfilled? Has God forgotten to be gracious, has he in anger withheld his mercies? "Has his right hand," I said, "lost its grasp? Does it hang powerless, the arm of the Most High?" But then, O Lord, I call to mind thy deeds; I recall thy wonderful acts in times gone by. I meditate upon thy works and muse on all that thou hast done. (Ps 77:1-12 NEB)

Another psalmist tells us that weeping may tarry through the night, which literally translated means that it may come as "an overnight guest." But "joy comes with the morning" (Ps 30:5). As Christians, we celebrate Easter morning with hallelujahs because Jesus Christ is alive. His living presence calls to you and to me and says, "Come, find authentic life." He is alive. Come, share in his aliveness. Walk in the light as he is the Light. We have the assurance that the darkness will never master his light. In him is life and light to guide us through the darkness, valleys, and difficult days.

In your mind's eye picture yourself as you were as a child, small and helpless. You open a strange door in front of you and step into a dark room. The door closes behind you with a bang. You are frightened. You look around and try to peer through the blackness, but you cannot see anything. Your heart begins to beat with fear. You start to cry. The dark shadows are filled with terror. You are frozen motionless. Suddenly, the door swings open. You recognize your father in the light that falls into the room. You run to him, and he picks you up in his arms and holds you close. Now you feel secure, and your anxiety subsides.

Putting our hand in the hand of Christ, we turn and walk into the darkness, assured that he will walk with us into the light that lies beyond the darkness. Whether the journey through darkness is filled with silence or new songs to learn, I step with confidence beside the one for whom both light and darkness are the same.

Notes

[1]John Baillie, *And the Life Everlasting* (New York: Charles Scribner's Sons, 1933) 163.

[2]Pinchas Lapide, *The Resurrection of Jesus: A Jewish Perspective*, trans. Wilhelm C. Linns (Minneapolis MN: Augsburg Press, 1983) 54.

[3]Douglas John Hall, *Professing the Faith* (Minneapolis MN: Fortress Press, 1993) 359.

[4]Jürgen Moltmann, *Theology of Hope* (New York: Harper & Row, 1967) 165.

[5]Wolfhart Pannenberg, *The Apostles' Creed in the Light of Today's Questions* (Philadelphia: Westminster Press, 1972) 97.

[6]Norine Dicksen Campbell, *Patrick Henry: Patriot and Statesman* (New York: Devin-Adair Co., 1969) 417-18.

[7]Ibid., 418.